D1568709

Gastrointestinal Polyps

Dedication

We dedicate this book to our colleagues in gastroenterology
and our teachers in pathology.

Contents

Preface

With the advent of endoscopic techniques, the gastro-intestinal tract has now become more accessible to clinical investigators. Polyps are amongst the commoner lesions biopsied and/or removed at the time of gastrointestinal endoscopy. The term "Polyp" derives from the Greek for "multiple feet" (poly, many and pes, feet) or "little nipple". In current clinical practice a polyp is defined as *"a circumscribed protrusion above the mucosa, stalked or sessile"*[1]. The biological behaviour of a polyp relates entirely to its pathological nature; hence the importance of an accurate histological diagnosis.

There have been many advances in our understanding of the biological behaviour, clinical associations and the prevalence of gastrointestinal polyps. We believe that these justify a dedicated book on the subject. While many textbooks and atlases include them as part of gastrointestinal tumours, none have been so comprehensively devoted to the polyp as this heavily illustrated book. It is designed to be the complete companion; a bench book not only for the practising histopathologist who regularly examines oesophageal, gastric, duodenal and intestinal polyps as part of his/her daily work but also for the endoscopist who regularly biopsies them. It will aid readers in the identification of the commoner polyps. Furthermore, this book will allow the reader to recognise related diseases and be aware of the biological behaviour of polyps without having to refer continuously to the standard textbooks in which this type of information is widely scattered.

The layout of the book has been designed sequentially to describe the commoner synonyms when appropriate, the prevalence, endoscopic/macroscopic appearances and microscopic features followed by a section on the biological behaviour and associated conditions. There is a section on treatment, if applicable, with a list of key references.

The classification is broadly modelled on the recent WHO recent classification in an attempt to reduce the potential confusion by use of differing appellations.

1. Maratka Z. In: Terminology, Definitions and Diagnostic Criteria in Digestive Endoscopy, 2nd Edition. Ed. English Version Colin-Jones DG. Pub. Normed Verlag. Bad Homburg.1989, p27.

Najib Y Haboubi
Karel Geboes
Neil A Shepherd
Ian C Talbot

November 2001

Contributors

Karel Geboes, MD, PhD
Professor of Pathology
Specialist in Internal Medicine and Pathology
Department of Pathology
University Hospitals K U Leuven
Belgium

Nadine Ectors, MD, PhD
Associate Professor of Pathology
Department of Pathology
University Hospitals K U Leuven
Belgium

Najib Y Haboubi, MB ChB, DPath, FRCPath
Head of Surgical Pathology
Trafford General Hospital
Formerly Head of Pathology
University Hospital of South Manchester
UK

Neil A Shepherd, MB, BS, FRCPath
Professor of Pathology
Consultant Histopathologist and Head of Department
Gloucestershire Royal Hospital
Gloucester, UK

Ian C Talbot, MB, BS, MD, FRCPath
Professor of Pathology and
Consultant Histopathologist
Academic Department of Pathology
St Mark's Hospital
Harrow, UK

Acknowledgements

We would like to acknowledge all those people who have helped us in preparing this book, particularly our colleagues in gastro-enterology and pathology, specifically Professors G. D'Haens, A. Gevers, T. Warnes, G. T. Williams and Doctors H. Ali, R. Gardy, P. Miller and N. Safarani for providing a large number of the illustrations in this book. We would also like to acknowledge the team of the Medical Illustration Department at the University Hospital of South Manchester for their help and one of our sons, Omar, who has spent a long time helping in the organisation of the manuscripts.

Polyps of the Oesophagus

Oesophageal polyps
Normal structure
Glycogenic acanthosis
Heterotopic sebaceous glands
Squamous cell papillomas
Viral warts
Polypoidal dysplasia
Inflammatory polyps
Fibrous polyps
Leiomyomas
Granular cell tumours
Polypoidal squamous cell carcinomas
Polypoidal adenocarcinoma
Malignant melanoma
Neurogenic tumours

K Geboes

OESOPHAGEAL POLYPS

Introduction

Whilst oesophageal cancer remains one of the leading causes of cancer mortality, oesophageal polyps are relatively unusual, compared with polyps in other parts of the gastrointestinal tract. From both a clinical and a pathological point of view, polyps of the oesophagus may be divided into two main groups, intramural and intraluminal growths. The vast majority of the intramural tumours are stromal tumours. They are made up of variable proportions of smooth muscle and fibrous tissue. Such intraluminal polypoidal growths usually originate in the submucosa and are covered by normal squamous epithelium. Endoscopic biopsies usually fail to reveal the nature of both intramural and intraluminal tumours except for those lesions that have originated from the epithelium. Oesophageal cancer rarely presents itself as a polypoid lesion.

NORMAL STRUCTURE

The oesophagus can be grossly divided into four segments. The distances given are measured from the incisor teeth.

- The cervical oesophagus extends from the cricoid cartilage (15 cm) to the level of the thoracic inlet (suprasternal notch) (18 cm).

- The upper thoracic segment comprises that part between the thoracic inlet and the tracheal bifurcation (24 cm).

- The mid-thoracic segment extends to the level of the eighth thoracic vertebra (32 cm).

- The lower thoracic segment extends to the junction with the stomach (40 cm) and includes the abdominal oesophagus.

The International Union against Cancer proposed this division into four segments for the purposes of classification, staging and reporting of oesophageal malignancy. In anatomical textbooks the oesophagus is divided into three segments: the cervical oesophagus extending to the level of T2–T3, the thoracic and the abdominal oesophagus. The anatomical landmarks supporting this division are not as well defined. Moreover, the anatomical regions for the oesophagus are not fixed: in fact they merge into each other and vary with age.[1,2]

The gastro-oesophageal junction can be defined anatomically, microscopically and physiologically. Endoscopic landmarks are the upper margin of the diaphragmatic indentation and the proximal margin of the gastric folds. The mucosal junction does not correspond to the muscular junction as defined by the proximal edge of the gastric folds[3] and normally lies within 2 cm of the muscular junction. Endoscopically the squamocolumnar junction is easily recognisable as an irregular line: the Z-line. The gastric mucosa is red-orange in colour and the oesophageal mucosa is pale with fine blood vessels.

The oesophageal mucosa

Histologically, the oesophageal mucosa consists of non-keratinising, stratified squamous epithelium, lamina propria and muscularis mucosae (Fig 1.1). The deep border of the epithelium is irregular due to the presence of transitory folds and high conical papillae of highly vascularised connective tissue. The epithelium can be divided into several compartments or zones: the basal zone, the intermediate (or prickle cell) zone and the superficial zone. This division corresponds with the processes of cell renewal, proliferation, differentiation (or maturation) and cell death that occur within the epithelium.

The basal zone is composed of one layer at the junction with the underlying stroma (in which the proliferative compartment resides) and two or three layers above containing immature cells. A periodic acid-Schiff (PAS) stain will demonstrate the upper extent of these glycogen-poor basal cells. Above the basal zone the intermediate and superficial layers consist of glycogen-rich cells that become progressively flatter towards the surface. In the basal cell layer melanocytes and endocrine cells may be present. Non-epithelial cells that are normally present within the epithelium are lymphocytes, Langerhans cells and occasional basophils.[3–5]

At the lower end of the oesophagus there is a sudden change from stratified squamous epithelium to mucin-secreting columnar epithelium.

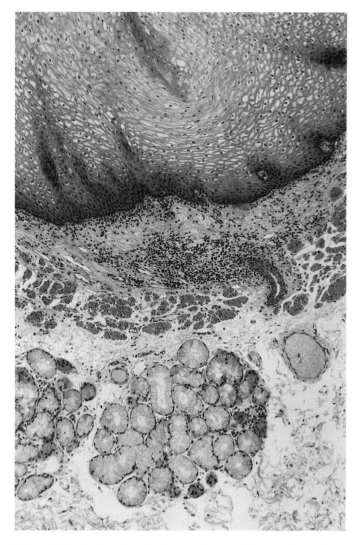

Figure 1.1 – Section through the upper layers of the oesophagus showing the typical non-keratinised squamous epithelium and the subjacent submucosa containing an oesophageal mucus-secreting gland.

Oesophageal glands

Cardiac-type glands are found in 6–16% of oesophagi. They are diffusely scattered in the lamina propria through all levels of the oesophagus and open directly into the lumen through ducts lined by gastric foveolar-like cells. They have been considered to be normal constituents, embryological remnants and heterotopias.

Located in the submucosa are typical tubulo-alveolar glands that resemble salivary glands. Each gland consists of a number of lobules (composed of acini and ducts) and is connected to the mucosal surface by a duct, which is roughly vertical. The duct is lined by stratified epithelium near the oesophageal lumen and by a flattened cuboidal epithelium at the junction with the acini. The acini are composed of mucus (chief) and serous (subsidiary) secreting cells as well as myoepithelial cells.[5]

GLYCOGENIC ACANTHOSIS

Prevalence

With the combined use of endoscopy and barium studies, glycogenic acanthosis can be seen in 25% of the adult population.[6,7] It can also be seen in up to 15% of upper endoscopies.

Endoscopic appearance

- They appear to be plaque-like and occur predominantly in the lower oesophagus.

- They are slightly elevated, white, round or oval, smooth surfaced lesions (Fig 1.2).

- Most lesions are under 5 mm in diameter, although lesions up to 1.5 cm in diameter have been reported.

- If extensive, the lesions may coalesce to form larger plaques (Fig 1.3). These plaques show no associated hyperaemia or oedema.

Microscopic features

There is usually thickening of the epithelium with elongation of the papillae due to hypertrophy of squamous cells, in particular those of the intermediate layer (Fig 1.4). The cellular enlargement is caused by the accumulation of abundant glycogen. This gives the cells their characteristic pale or vacuolated appearance. There is no cellular atypia, keratosis or associated inflammation. They should not be confused with moniliasis.

Biological behaviour and associated conditions

They should be considered as a variant of normal and are asymptomatic. There is no defined relationship with infection or malignancy.

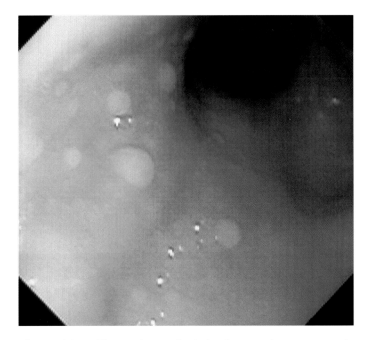

Figure 1.2 – Glycogenic acanthosis in the oesophagus commonly appears as shallow, white, round, smooth discrete elevations.

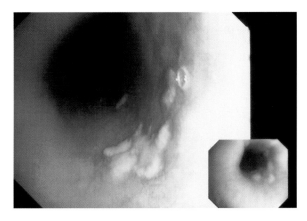

Figure 1.3 – In extensive glycogenic acanthosis the lesions may coalesce to form larger plaques.

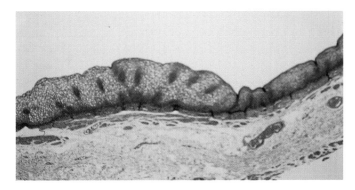

Figure 1.4 – A case of glycogenic acanthosis. Note the regular thickening of the epithelium due to the presence of enlarged cells, with glycogen rich clear cytoplasm. There is no cellular atypia.

Management

No specific treatment is required.

HETEROTOPIC SEBACEOUS GLANDS

Prevalence

These are rare lesions. In one autopsy series they were found at different levels in 2% of the cases.[8]

Endoscopic appearance

- They appear as yellow-grey, plaque-like, oval and rounded lesions, 1–5 mm in dimension, sometimes there are several present (Fig 1.5).

- They should be distinguished from the more common glycogenic acanthosis.

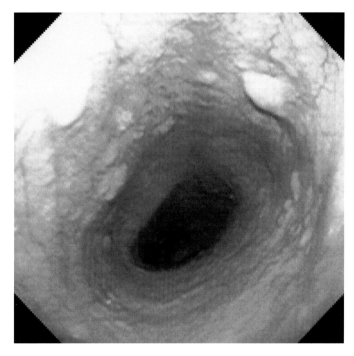

Figure 1.5 – Heterotopic sebaceous glands can appear as grey, plaque-like, slightly elevated lesions. Sometimes there are several present as shown in this case.

Microscopic feature

These lesions are characterised by the presence of mature sebaceous glands deep in the oesophageal mucosa.

Biological behaviour and associated conditions

They are invariably benign and not associated with defined conditions.

Management

No specific treatment required.

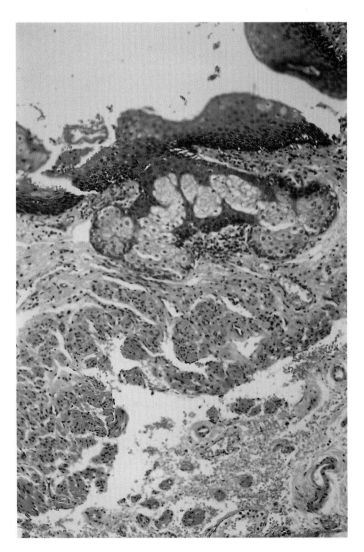

Figure 1.6 – Low power photograph showing mature sebaceous glands deep in the oesophageal epithelium.

SQUAMOUS CELL PAPILLOMAS

Prevalence

These are rare lesions with an estimated prevalence of 14:100 000.[9] Only two lesions were found in series of 19 982 post-mortems and three and six cases were reported from series with 6157 and 14 900 endoscopic examinations, respectively.[10,11]

The age range of patients with papilloma varies from 14 to 78, with a mean age of 54 years. About 75% of the reported cases have been in males. The lesion is less common in children.[12] A giant form and a form of oesophageal papillomatosis have been described but both are extremely rare.[13]

Endoscopic appearance

- Squamous cell papillomas may be located in any region of the oesophagus, but there is a strong predilection for the distal oesophagus.

- They appear as smooth, round, pink, sharply demarcated, sessile tumours (Fig 1.7). These vary in size from 0.4 to 1.5 cm.

- They are generally single but multiple papillomata may occur (Fig 1.8).

- A variant of oesophageal papillomatosis is characterised by the occurrence of multiple confluent papillomas with a verrucous pattern (resembling verrucous carcinoma) (Fig 1.9).

Microscopic features

The papillary architecture consists of finger-like projections of delicate fibrous tissue covered by acanthotic stratified squamous epithelium (Fig 1.10). The epithelium is organised in the same manner as normal oesophageal mucosa and shows the normal differentiation from the basal to the surface layers and lacks atypia.

In oesophageal papillomatosis, atypia and inflammatory features may be present.

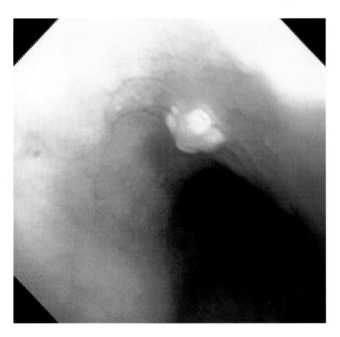

Figure 1.7 – Endoscopic appearance of a solitary small squamous papilloma of the oesophagus. The surface is slightly irregular. The lesion is well demarcated.

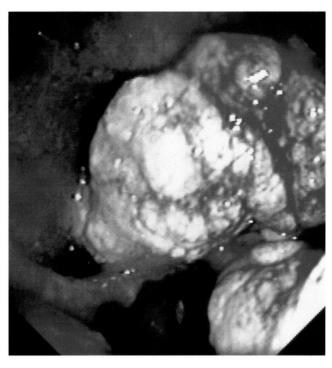

Figure 1.9 – Endoscopic picture of a (giant) oesophageal papillomatosis, a rare condition, characterised by the presence of a large sessile lesion.

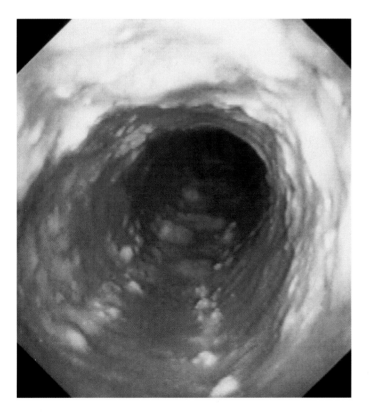

Figure 1.8 – Squamous papilloma of the oesophagus is usually a single lesion. Occasionally, multiple lesions are present as seen in this case.

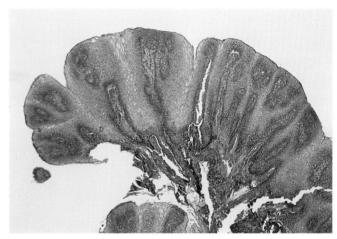

Figure 1.10 – Low power photograph showing the fingerlike projections of the fibrovascular core of a squamous oesophageal papilloma. The surface epithelium is mature and lacks cellular atypia.

Biological behaviour and associated conditions

There is no evidence of an association with malignancy.

The human papilloma virus (HPV) antigen (mainly types 16 and 18) has been identified in up to 50% of tissues tested using immunoperoxidase and by *in situ* hybridisation, but is less common in other series.[14,15] Papillomatosis can recur and may be associated with malignancy. It may however differ aetiologically from the solitary small squamous cell papilloma.[16] The distinction between papillomatosis and viral wart is unclear. Aetiologically there are probably differences because of the association with HPV or even the type of HPV involved. Some of the small papillomas or polypoid lesions in the distal oesophagus are associated with gastro-oesophageal reflux disease. Furthermore, similar macroscopic lesions can be identified in asymptomatic patients.

It appears that what is observed endoscopically as a small papillomatous lesion in the distal oesophagus is a lesion with several different possible aetiologies, such as viral or reflux disease. The precise aetiology cannot always be established.

Rare forms of oesophageal papillomatosis

Papillomatosis of the oesophagus is reportedly associated with a rare congenital syndrome (Goltz–Gorlin syndrome). This consists of congenital poikiloderma with keratoconus and skeletal and tooth defects.[17] Patients with acanthosis nigricans may, rarely, develop a very fine papilloma-like nodularity of the oesophagus.

Management

Endoscopic resection is an adequate treatment. Recurrence is not reported for small squamous cell papillomas.

Papillomatosis may be treated by local endoscopic injection with anti-viral drugs.[18]

VIRAL WARTS

Synonyms

Condyloma.

Prevalence

Squamous cell papillomas associated with human papilloma virus are uncommon. They occur mainly in children and are similar to, and usually associated with, similar lesions in the larynx, the trachea and occasionally in the bronchi.[19]

Endoscopic appearance

- Lesions vary from a few millimetres to 1 cm in diameter.

- They appear as pale, broad-based excrescences.

- They are often multiple and usually found in the mid-oesophagus although the entire oesophagus may be affected.[19]

Microscopic features

These lesions are essentially made up of a fibrovascular core of lamina propria with a hyperplastic overlying epithelium lacking atypia and keratinisation (Fig 1.11).

Koilocytes may or may not be present.

The distinction between squamous papilloma and squamous papilloma associated with the human papilloma virus (viral wart) is not always clear.

Biological behaviour and associated conditions

They are usually found incidentally.

Spontaneous resolution may occur and in general, squamous papillomas behave in a benign manner.

Management

Endoscopic removal is sufficient as treatment. No follow-up is needed.

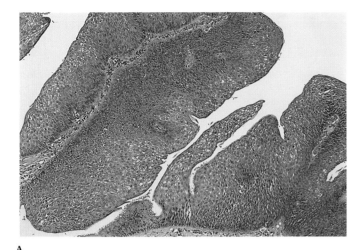

A

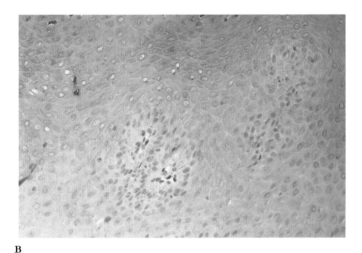

B

Figure 1.11 – (A) A photomicrograph of a viral wart. There is a fibrovascular core covered by a thickened papillary squamous layer. Koilocytosis. (B) In situ hybridisation shows a positive reaction for HPV 6–11.

POLYPOIDAL DYSPLASIA

Synonyms

Adenomatous neoplasm, adenoma, adenomatous changes, adenomatous hyperplasia, nodular dysplasia, dysplasia associated lesion or mass (DALM).

Prevalence

Adenomas with the morphological features of a tubular or villous adenoma are rarely seen in the distal oesophagus. In fact the only convincing examples that have been documented have occurred in the columnar-lined (Barrett's) oesophagus.[20–22]

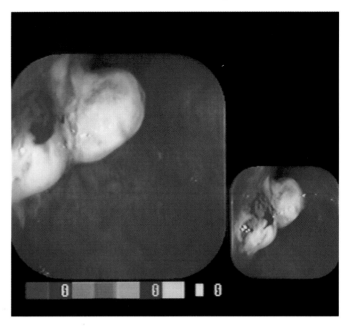

Figure 1.12 – An endoscopic picture of a polypoidal lesion arising in a background of Barrett's oesophagus.

In general we believe that the term adenoma, as applied to the oesophagus, is a misnomer. Such lesions are best designated polypoid dysplasia in columnar lined (Barrett's) oesophagus.

Endoscopic appearance

- These lesions usually appear as irregular and elevated masses (Fig 1.12).

- The size varies from a few millimetres to 1 cm in diameter, occasionally larger.

Microscopic features

These lesions can appear as rather polypoid areas of glandular metaplasia and dysplasia in Barrett's oesophagus (Fig 1.13).

The surface and glands are lined by a single layer of columnar cells. These cells show features of specialised intestinal epithelium, sometimes in a mosaic with other types of metaplasia (as is commonly seen in Barrett's oesophagus).

The columnar cells may show features of dysplasia with loss of mucin secretion, the presence of elongated, basally

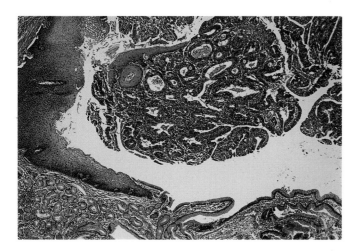

Figure 1.13 – Microscopy of an oesophageal glandular polypoid lesion occurring in Barrett's oesophagus with features of an adenoma.

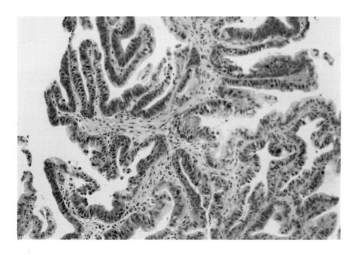

Figure 1.14 – This shows a case of villous adenomatous polypoidal dysplasia in Barrett's oesophagus. Note the adenomatous configuration of the lesion and the severe cellular atypia of the columnar epithelium.

located nuclei and a tendency to palisading (Fig 1.14). Dysplastic areas can be mixed with hyperplastic appearing glands.

It should be noted that rare examples of submucosal adenomas have also been reported.[23]

Biological behaviour and associated conditions

The presence of a mass often implies an advanced stage of dysplasia that has a greater probability of being associated with invasive carcinoma.

Management

Endoscopic resection may be sufficient, provided that microscopic examination reveals no foci of invasive changes.

INFLAMMATORY POLYPS

Synonyms

Oesophagogastric polyp, inflammatory reflux polyp, oesophagogastric polyp-fold complex.

Prevalence

Not precisely known.

Endoscopic appearance

- Characteristically these appear as a solitary small sessile polypoid lesion occurring at or near the gastro-oesophageal junction (Fig 1.15). Less commonly they can appear as multiple small sessile polypoid lesions.

- Endoscopically the lesions are round.

- They vary from 5–20 mm in diameter, with a smooth and erythematous surface, often with a small superficial erosion on the top.

- Endoscopic features of oesophagitis are often found.

- There may be a prominent fold of mucosa (a sentinel fold) leading up to the polyp from the gastro-oesophageal junction.[24–26]

Microscopic features

The typical features are a mixture of granulation tissue and inflammation of the lamina propria covered by squamous epithelium showing features of basal hyperplasia, with varying erosion of the epithelium and often marked active inflammatory cell infiltrate (Fig 1.16). Sometimes the polyp

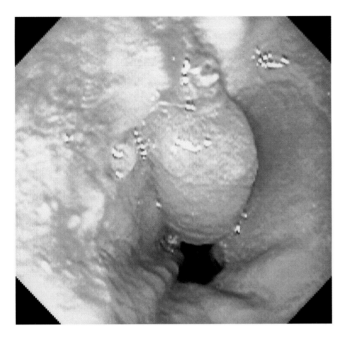

Figure 1.15 – Endoscopic picture of an oesophageal inflammatory polyp. The lesion is usually round with a smooth, slightly irregular and erythematous surface and is usually seen at the lower end of the oesophagus.

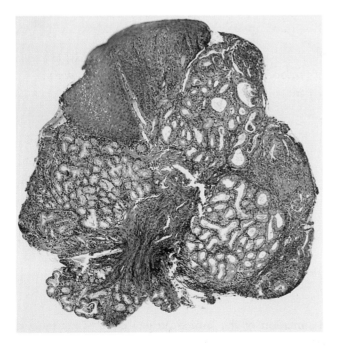

Figure 1.16 – A case of an inflammatory polyp of the oesophagus, which is lined in part by granulation tissue, in part by orderly squamous epithelium and in part by columnar epithelium.

is partially covered by junctional columnar epithelium. The adjacent oesophageal mucosa is usually inflamed.

Biological behaviour and associated conditions

Inflammatory polyps develop mostly in patients with a hiatus hernia and/or with reflux oesophagitis. They can also occur in patients without such a history and in patients with other less common causes of oesophagitis.[27]

They are entirely benign. In the past, several of these have been erroneously reported as squamous cell papilloma.[28]

Management

No treatment is needed, except for the associated oesophagitis.

FIBROUS POLYPS

Synonyms

Fibrovascular polyp, fibroma, fibromyxoma, fibrolipoma, lipoma, pedunculated lipoma.

Prevalence

These are rare lesions. In larger autopsy series the incidence of benign non-epithelial oesophageal tumours is usually less than 0.25%. In some series the incidence of fibrovascular polyps is second to smooth muscle tumours. It is most likely that inflammatory polyps are not included in such studies because they are too small and may not be visible at post-mortem. The majority of patients with fibrous polyps are middle-aged to elderly with males being more frequently affected.

Endoscopic and gross appearance

- Smooth surfaced elongated intraluminal masses that are usually more or less pedunculated (Fig 1.17).

- The majority arise in the upper oesophagus, in the region of the cricoid.

- They are often quite large. In approximately 75% of the reported cases the lesions have been over 7 cm in length. A number of cases were reported where the mass was over 20 cm in length, sometimes extending for almost the entire length of the oesophagus. The larger lesions tend to be more or less located distally. Moreover, even when large, they may be missed endoscopically because their surface is usually similar to normal oesophageal mucosa.

- Rare instances of multiple fibrovascular or double-pedunculated polyps have been reported.[29,30]

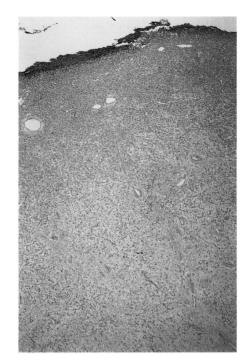

Figure 1.18 – Microscopic picture of an oesophageal fibrous polyp showing ulcerated surface epithelium and abundant underlying fibrous stroma.

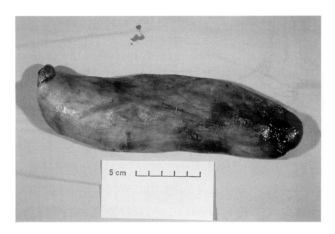

Figure 1.17 – Surgical specimen of an oesophageal fibrous polyp. These are usually large, pedunculated lesions with a smooth surface.

Microscopic features

They consist of fibrous tissue (which may be myxomatous) with thin–walled blood vessels (Figs 1.18 & 1.19).

Sometimes a variable amount of adipose tissue is present and this can be the predominant component.

The mucosa is usually, but not always, intact.

Biological behaviour and associated conditions

They are essentially benign. Very few cases have been reported in which epithelial malignancy has developed.

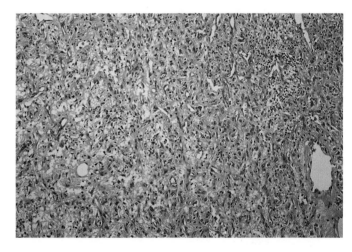

Figure 1.19 – In this high power view fibrovascular proliferation can be seen with few chronic inflammatory cells.

Occasionally rapid growth has been noted but this is probably the result of torsion and oedema.[31]

The patient may have minimal symptoms, but may present with dysphagia or vomiting after meals and regurgitation. In a few cases, the tumour itself regurgitates into the mouth or even outside.

Respiratory symptoms, such as wheezing from tracheal compression, choking and haematemesis, may occasionally occur.

Management

Complete removal of the lesion, either surgically or endoscopically, is indicated. The site of the polyp and its volume define the method of resection.[32,33]

LEIOMYOMAS

Synonyms

Gastrointestinal stromal tumours, smooth muscle tumours.

Prevalence

Leiomyomas are the most common non-epithelial tumours of the oesophagus. Most oesophageal leiomyomas are tiny, subclinical lesions. They have been designated as 'seedling leiomyomas' and occur in up to 10% of adult oesophagi.[34] Larger lesions are less common. They occur more frequently in males with a ratio of 2–3:1. Patients are usually in their fifth decade. It is rare in childhood.[35]

Endoscopic appearance

- Occasionally leiomyomas present as pedunculated or sessile intraluminal tumours. These can be removed endoscopically.

- 97% of cases present as intramural tumours (Fig 1.20) at endoscopy, demonstrating a well circumscribed, curved or rounded indentation of the oesophageal wall with a free mobile overlying intact mucosa. Biopsy is contraindicated in such cases, since diagnostic material is rarely obtained and subsequent surgical enucleation is made more difficult. Biopsy may be indicated if irregularity or ulceration are present, which suggest malignancy.

- Leiomyomas are generally single tumours. Only 2–3% of patients present with two or more. Symptomatic tumours are of moderate size, from 2–5 cm.

- Although they may occur anywhere in the oesophagus, more than 50% of the lesions are found in the lower third.

- They arise more commonly in the circular muscle layer.

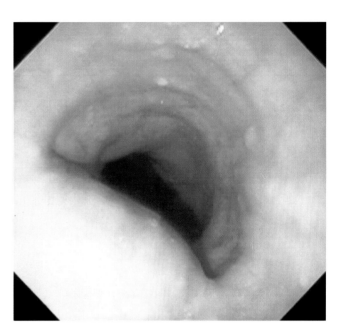

Figure 1.20 – Endoscopic picture of an oesophageal leiomyoma. The lesion is located intramurally. The oesophageal wall is elevated but retains a smooth overlying mucosa.

Microscopic features

The lesions are composed of interlacing bundles of smooth muscle cells that may show hypertrophy of the individual cells (Fig 1.21).

Necrosis and central ulceration are usually absent.

Vascularity is not prominent.

Mitoses are absent or extremely rare.

Calcification has been reported to occur in less than 2% of cases.

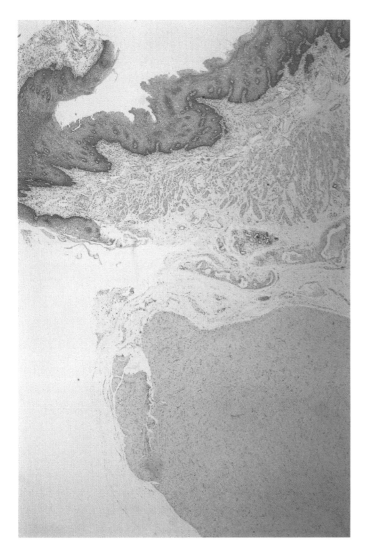

Figure 1.21 – Microscopic picture of an oesophageal leiomyoma, covered by normal epithelium.

They usually show a positive reaction to antibodies directed against the smooth muscle actin and can be positive for CD34, a sialylated transmembrane glycoprotein in endothelial cells and myeloid progenitor cells, which can be positive in gastrointestinal, spindle cell type and stromal tumours. Oesophageal gastrointestinal stromal tumours (GISTs) show mutations for c-kit and can be identified with immunohistochemical techniques that use antibodies directed against c-kit. Compared to oesophageal leiomyomas, genuine oesophageal GISTs occur in an older population (median age 63 years), but, as for the leiomyoma group, men predominate. It is important to distinguish between oesophageal leiomyomas and GISTs because the latter group have a high risk of malignant behaviour.[36]

Biological behaviour and associated conditions

Most cases of oesophageal stromal tumours with smooth muscle differentiation are benign. Malignant cases (leiomyosarcomas) are extremely rare.

Management

Management may be facilitated by endoscopic ultrasonography. This allows the exact location and extent of the tumour to be determined.[37] Surgical enucleation or a conservative approach[38] are most commonly advocated for these lesions.

GRANULAR CELL TUMOURS

Synonyms

Granular cell myoblastomas, granular cell neurofibromas, Abrikosoff's tumours.

Prevalence

These are rare lesions with just over 100 cases reported in the literature. The mean age of patients is about 40 years.

There is no significant sex preponderance for granular cell tumours of the oesophagus and the majority of patients are asymptomatic.

Endoscopic appearance

- The lesion usually appears as a raised, firm, yellowish nodule with a smooth surface covered by fairly normal mucosa (Fig 1.22). Some cases have presented as an annular constriction.

- In general they measure under 1–2 cm in diameter but larger tumours causing obstructive symptoms have been reported.

- In more than 50% of the cases they are located in the lower third of the oesophagus.

- They are usually solitary, although examples of multiple lesions have been reported.

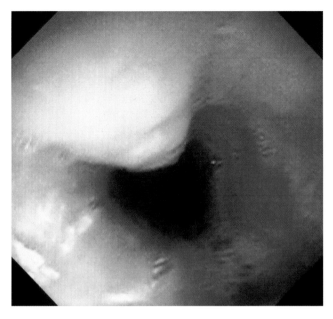

Figure 1.22 – Endoscopic appearance of a granular cell tumour of the oesophagus. The lesion appears as a raised, firm nodule covered with smooth surface.

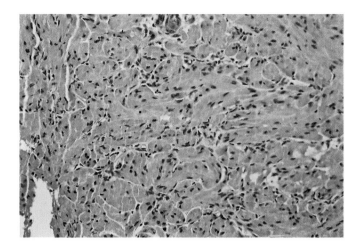

Figure 1.24 – A higher power view of a case of granular cell tumour. The cells characteristically have small pyknotic nuclei and eosinophilic cytoplasm.

Microscopic features

These tumours consist of plump cells with a granular eosinophilic cytoplasm and small centrally or peripherally located nuclei (Fig 1.23 & 1.24).

The granules can be stained using the PAS reaction (after prior diastase digestion) and also stains with S100 protein.

The overlying squamous epithelium may show prominent hyperplasia, which can be mistaken for infiltrating squamous cell carcinoma, particularly in superficial biopsies.[39]

Biological behaviour and associated conditions

These are benign lesions. Only one case with malignant behaviour has been reported.[40]

Management

Endoscopic removal (when feasible) or surgical enucleation.

POLYPOIDAL SQUAMOUS CELL CARCINOMA

Prevalence

Carcinoma of the oesophagus is largely a disease of late middle to old age.

The death rate from oesophageal cancer varies greatly in different countries and regions.

The highest incidence is reported in the black population of South Africa.

In Europe, the highest incidence is found in France.

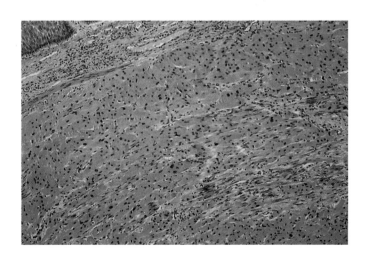

Figure 1.23 – Microscopic appearance of an oesophageal granular cell tumour. There are sheets of cells with a monotonous bland appearance.

Endoscopic and gross appearance

- Oesophageal carcinoma is often discovered at a late stage.

- Advanced carcinoma is usually a nodular lesion with varying degrees of ulceration (Fig 1.25).

- Polypoid tumour without ulceration is extremely rare.

- There are two other types of polypoidal squamous cell carcinoma, namely the verrucous and the spindle cell variants. Both are usually exophytic large tumours.

- Early oesophageal carcinoma is a tumour that has not extended beyond the submucosa. It can present grossly as either occult, erosive, plaque or papillary types. The latter lesion has a papillary or polypoid configuration, usually 1–3 cm in diameter. There is a clear demarcation between the edge of the lesion and the surrounding normal mucosa. On occasion erosions are present on the surface. Early oesophageal cancer of this type is rare.[41,42]

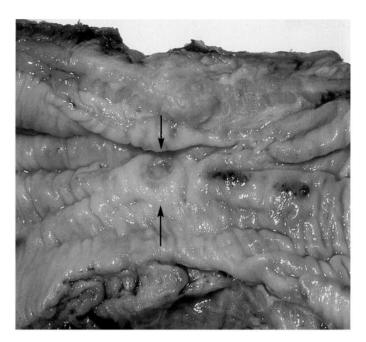

Figure 1.25 – A surgical specimen showing a partly ulcerated and partly raised tumour.

Microscopic features

Well differentiated carcinoma shows keratinisation and large polygonal or round cancer cells. Moderate differentiation is characterised by round, oval or polygonal cells with a certain amount of polymorphism (Fig 1.26). There may be moderate keratinisation or a few epithelial pearls. Poorly differentiated types are composed of spindle-shaped, ovoid, or irregular cells that are usually small with scanty cytoplasm. Mitoses are frequent. There is little or no keratinisation. Spindle cell carcinoma is a variant of squamous cell carcinoma with a polypoid appearance and histologically either a pure spindle cell component (pseudosarcoma) or mixed spindle and epithelial components (carcinosarcoma).

Verrucous carcinoma is another rare variant with papillary growth and well differentiated histology. Similar tumours occur in other sites of the body like the oral cavity, larynx, external genitalia and anal canal.

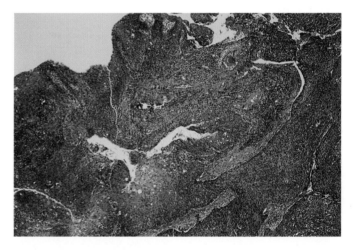

Figure 1.26 – Microscopic picture of a polypoidal moderately differentiated squamous cell carcinoma.

Biological behaviour and associated conditions

Five year survival rates are poor, except for patients with an early oesophageal carcinoma.

On the other hand, verrucous carcinoma has a better prognosis because this is a slow growing tumour with a late metastatic potential.[43]

Management

Surgical treatment may be combined with adjuvant chemo- and radiotherapy. However, in some series the results of radical surgery may be similar to those in patients treated by radiotherapy alone. This reflects the usually advanced stage at the time of presentation.

POLYPOIDAL ADENOCARCINOMA

Synonyms

Mucus secreting carcinomas.

Prevalence

The incidence and prevalence have not yet been determined. Based on the available data it is estimated that the prevalence of adenocarcinoma in patients with Barrett's oesophagus amounts to 10%.[44]

Adenocarcinoma involving the oesophagus usually occur in the distal third.

Most adenocarcinoma is associated with Barrett's oesophagus, either long or short-segment disease. Gastro-oesophageal junction carcinomas behave clinically like Barrett's adenocarcinoma.

Endoscopic and gross appearance

- The gross appearance is variable. Advanced tumours usually present as large, ulcerated, fungating, polypoid or diffusely infiltrating masses (Fig 1.27).

- Early adenocarcinoma is usually flat but some may be polypoid.

Microscopic features

The microscopic features (Fig 1.28) are similar to those of gastric adenocarcinoma.

Most tumours are well or moderately differentiated adenocarcinoma.

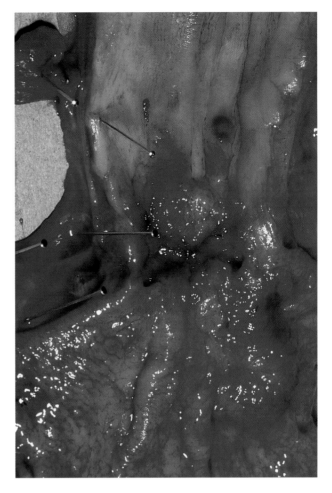

Figure 1.27 – Surgical specimen of an oesophageal adenocarcinoma showing a part polypoid and part ulcerated appearance.

The diffuse infiltrative type with signet-ring cells is less common.

Since most cases arise on a background of Barrett's oesophagus, islands of Barrett's type epithelium are usually seen showing different grades of dysplasia.[45]

Biological behaviour and associated conditions

Overall prognosis is poor except for early oesophageal adenocarcinoma.

Management

Surgery may be combined with adjuvant chemo- or radiotherapy.

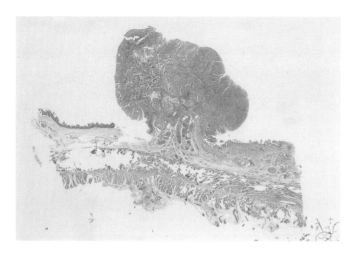

Figure 1.28 – Low power microphotograph of a polypoid oesophageal adenocarcinoma.

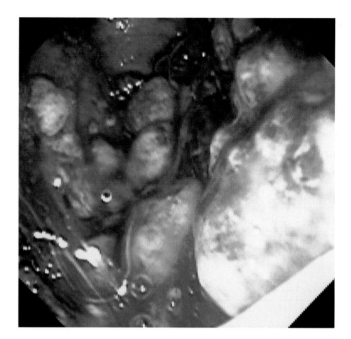

Figure 1.29 – Endoscopic picture of a primary melanoma of the oesophagus presenting as a large, pigmented, polypoid lesion.

MALIGNANT MELANOMA

Synonyms

Melanosarcoma, melanocarcinoma.

Prevalence

Extremely rare lesion with, to date, about 130 documented cases published.

Patients are usually in their sixth to eighth decade.

Men outnumber women by 2 to 1.[46]

Endoscopic appearance

- The lesion is generally located in the middle or lower third.

- It presents as a pigmented or non-pigmented, large polypoid, lesion (Fig 1.29).

Microscopic features

It bears the same characteristic features as those of melanoma in other sites.

The tumour is composed of uniform, poorly adhesive, pleomorphic cells (Fig 1.30) with variable amounts of pigment present. Junctional activity may be present in the adjacent squamous epithelium.

Some cases are associated with melanosis of the oesophageal mucosa.[47]

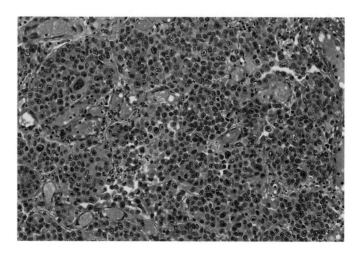

Figure 1.30 – In this case of oesophageal melanoma the cell population is composed of poorly adhesive, pleomorphic cells.

Biological behaviour and associated conditions

Poor prognosis with a mean survival time of 7 months.

Management

Surgery is the favoured treatment with palliative or curative intent.

Radiotherapy, chemotherapy and immunostimulation serve mainly as palliative or adjunctive measures.[48]

NEUROGENIC TUMOURS

Prevalence

Extremely rare. Only a few genuine cases of oesophageal schwannoma have been reported. One case presented as a giant oesophageal polyp and another as a solitary oesophageal schwannoma.[49,50]

Endoscopic appearance

- Schwannomas can present as giant intraluminal polyps, as rather flat, smooth-surfaced nodules or as a combination of both (Fig 1.31).

Microscopic features

Schwannomas appear as nodules showing a diffuse, fascicular growth pattern of spindle-shaped cells.

Nuclear palisading and vague Verocay body formation may be present.

Occasionally the lesion appears as a plexiform schwannoma. Immunohistochemistry with antibodies directed against the S100 protein and ultrastructural studies can confirm the nature of the lesion (Fig 1.32).

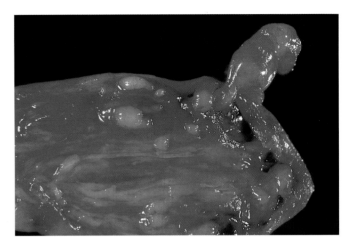

Figure 1.31 – Surgical specimen showing a plexiform schwannoma of the upper oesophagus, which appears as a pedunculated polyp and many flat, yellowish nodules.

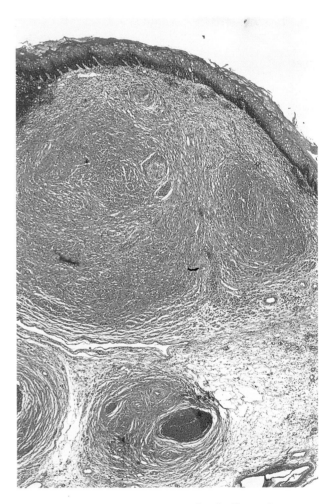

Figure 1.32 – Microscopic appearance of a plexiform schwannoma of the oesophagus. The lesion is composed of several vaguely encapsulated nodules of varying size, composed of fascieles of spindle-shaped cells.

Biological behaviour

Usually benign. Dysphagia and odynophagia may be the presenting symptoms.

Management

Surgery is usually advised.

REFERENCES

1. Hermanek P, Sobin LJ: *International Union Against Cancer (UICC) TNM Atlas Classification of Malignant tumours*, 3rd edn, 2nd Revision. Berlin: Springer-Verlag 1992

2. Maratka Z: Oesophagoscopie. In *Terminologie, Définitions et Criteres Diagnostiques en Endoscopie Digestive*, Maratka Z, Bader JP (eds). Bad Homburg, Normed Verlag 1990: pp. 34–35

3. DeNardi FG, Riddell RH: Oesophagus. In *Histology for Pathologists*, Sternberg SS (ed.). New York, Raven Press 1992: pp. 515–532

4. Geboes K: When is the esophageal mucosa normal? In *The oesophageal mucosa. 300 questions, 300 answers*, Giuli R, Tytgat GNJ, DeMeester TR, Galmiche JP (eds). Amsterdam, Elsevier 1994: pp. 21–28

5. Hopwood D: The oesophageal lining. In *Gastrointestinal and Oesophageal Pathology*, 2nd edn, Whitehead R (ed.). London, Churchill-Livingstone 1995: pp. 3–13

6. Blackstone MO: *Endoscopic Interpretation. Normal and Pathologic Appearances of the Gastrointestinal Tract*. New York, Raven Press 1984

7. Bender MD, Allison J, Cuartas F, Montgomery C: Glycogenic acanthosis of the oesophagus: a form of benign hyperplasia. *Gastroenterology* 1973; **65:** 373–380

8. De la Pava S, Pickren JW: Ectopic sebaceous glands in the oesophagus. *Arch Pathol* 1962; **73:** 397–399

9. Harrer WV, Sprague TH, Keeley FX: Squamous cell papilloma of the oesophagus. A case report and literature review. *J Med Soc HJ* 1975; **72:** 229–232

10. Plachta A: Benign tumours of the oesophagus – review of the literature and report of 99 cases. *Am J Gastroenterol* 1962; **38:** 639–651

11. Colina F, Solis JA, Munoz MT: Squamous papilloma of the oesophagus – a report of three cases and review of the literature. *Am J Gastroenterol* 1980; **74:** 410–414

12. Orlowska JR, Jarrosz D, Gugulski A, *et al*: Squamous cell papillomas of the oesophagus: report of 20 cases and literature review. *Am J Gastroenterol* 1994; **89:** 434–437

13. Walker JH: Giant papilloma of the thoracic oesophagus. *Am J Roentgenol* 1978; **131:** 519–520

14. Mastour M, Lefebvre A, Dambron P, *et al*: Papilloma oesophagien hémorrgigue associe a la prise d'anti-inflammatoires non steroidiens. *Gastroenterol Clin Biol* 1996; **20:** 406–407

15. Odze R, Antonioli D, Shocket D, *et al*: Oesophageal squamous papillomas. *Am J Surg Pathol* 1993; **17:** 803–812

16. Van Cutsem E, Geboes K, Visser L, *et al*: Squamous papillomatosis of the oesophagus with malignant degeneration and demonstration of the human papilloma virus. *Eur J Gastroenterol Hepatol* 1991; **3:** 561–566

17. Brinson RR, Schuman BM, Mills LR, *et al*: Multiple squamous papillomas of the oesophagus associated with Goltz syndrome. *Am J Gastroenterol* 1987; **82:** 1177–1179

18. Van Cutsem E, Snoeck R, Van Ranst M, *et al*: Successful treatment of a squamous papilloma of the hypopharynx-oesophagus by local injections of (S)-1-(3-hydroxy-2-phosphonylmethoxypropyl) cytosine. *J Med Vir* 1995; **45:** 230–235

19. Frootko NJ, Rogers JH: Oesophageal papillomata in the child. *J Laryngol Otol* 1978; **92:** 822–824

20. Whitehead R, Hamilton SR: Carcinoma and dysplasia in Barrett's oesophagus. In *Gastrointestinal and Oesophageal Pathology*, 2nd edn, Whitehead R (ed.). London, Churchill-Livingstone 1995, pp. 796–812

21. Haggitt RC: Barrett's oesophagus, dysplasia and adenocarcinoma. *Hum Pathol* 1994; **25:** 982–993

22. Ming SC: Adenocarcinoma and other epithelial tumours of the oesophagus. In *Pathology of the Gastrointestinal Tract*, Goldman H, Ming SC (eds). Philadelphia, WB Saunders Company 1992: pp. 459–477

23. Takubo K, Esaki Y, Watanabe A, *et al*: Adenoma accompanied by superficial squamous cell carcinoma of the oesophagus. *Cancer* 1993; **71:** 2435–2438

24. Rabin MS, Bremner CG, Botha JR: The reflux gastro-oesophageal polyp. *Am J Gastroenterol* 1980; **73:** 451–453

25. Styles RA, Gibb SP, Tarshis A, *et al*: Oesophago-gastric polyps: radiographic and endoscopic findings. *Radiology* 1985; **154:** 307–311

26. Van der Veer LD, Kramer K, Relkin R, Clearfield H: The oesophagogastric polyp-fold complex. *Am J Gastroenterol* 1984; **79:** 918–920

27. Ng FH, Wong SY, Chang CM, *et al*: Oesophageal actinomycosis: a case report. *Endoscopy* 1997; **29:** 133

28. Day DW, Dixon MF: Cysts, non-neoplastic polyps and tumours of the oesophagus. In *Biopsy Pathology of the Oesophagus, Stomach and Duodenum*, 2nd edn, Day DW, Dixon MF (eds). London, Chapman & Hall Medical 1995: pp. 50–61

29. Totten RS, Stout AP, Humphries GH, *et al*: Benign tumours and cysts of the oesophagus. *J Thorac Surg* 1953; **25:** 606–622

30. Burrell M, Toffler R: Fibrovascular polyp of the oesophagus. *Dig Dis* 1973; **18:** 714–718

31. Jang GC, Clouse ME, Fleischner FG: Fibrovascular polyp – a benign intraluminal tumour of the oesophagus. *Radiology* 1969; **92:** 1196–1200

32. Penagini R, Ranzi T, Velio P, *et al*: Giant fibrovascular polyp of the oesophagus: report of a case and effects on oesophageal function. *Gut* 1989; **30:** 1624–1629

33. Kise Y, Makunchi H, Shinada K, *et al*: Endoscopic resection indicated for double-pedunculated oesophageal lipoma. *Endoscopy* 1997; **29:** 131

34. Takubo K, Tsuchiya S, Nakagawa H: Seedling leiomyoma of the oesophagus and oesophagogastric junction zone. *Hum Pathol* 1981; **12:** 1006–1010

35. Seremetis MG, Lyoons WS, DeGuzman VC, Peabody JW Jr: Leiomyomata of the oesophagus: an analysis of 838 cases. *Cancer* 1976; **38:** 2166–2177

36. Miettinen M, Sarlomo-Rikala M, Sobin LH, Lasota J: Esophageal stromal tumors: a clinicopathologic, immunohistochemical and molecular genetic study of 17 cases and comparison with esophageal leiomyomas and leiomyosarcomas. *Am J Surg Pathol* 2000; **24:** 211–222

37. Tio TL, Tytgat GNJ, Den Hartog Jager FCA: Endoscopic ultrasonography for the evaluation of smooth muscle tumours of the upper gastrointestinal tract: an experience with 42 cases. *Gastrointest Endosc* 1990; **36:** 342–350

38. Cox MA, Cooper BT, Sagar G: Endoscopy and computed tomography in the diagnosis and follow-up of oesophageal leiomyoma. *Gut* 1995; **37:** 288–291

39. Johnston J, Helwig EB: Granular cell tumours of the gastrointestinal tract and perianal region. A study of 74 cases. *Dig Dis Sci* 1981; **26:** 807–816

40. Cone JB, Wetzel WJ: Oesophageal granular cell tumours. Report of two multicentric cases with observations on their natural histories. *J Surg Oncol* 1982; **20:** 14–16

41. Bogomoletz WV, Molas G, Gayet B, Potet F: Superficial squamous cell carcinoma of the esophagus. A report of 76 cases and review of the literature. *Am J Surg Pathol* 1989; **13:** 535–546

42. Endo M, Yamada A, Ide H, *et al*: Early cancer of the oesophagus: diagnosis and clinical evaluation. *Int Adv Surg Oncol* 1980; **3:** 49–71

43. Meyrowitz BR, Shea LT: The natural history of squamous verrucous carcinoma of the oesophagus. *J Thorac Cardiovasc Surg* 1971; **61:** 646–649

44. Li H: Malignant Barrett's oesophagus. *Eur J Cancer Prev* 1993; **2:** 47–52

45. Hamilton SR, Smith RRL, Cameron JL: Prevalence and characteristics of Barrett's oesophagus in patients with adenocarcinoma of the oesophagus or the oesophagogastric junction. *Hum Pathol* 1988; **19:** 942–948

46. Kreuser ED: Primary malignant melanoma of the oesophagus. *Virch Arch (A)* 1979; **385:** 49–59

47. Guzman RP, Wightman R, Ravinsky E, Unruh HW: Primary malignant melanoma of the oesophagus with diffuse melanocytic atypia and melanoma in-situ. *Am J Clin Pathol* 1989; **92:** 802–804

48. Isaacs JL, Quirke P: Two cases of primary malignant melanoma of the oesophagus. *Clin Radiol* 1988; **39:** 455–457

49. Eberelein TJ, Hannan R, Josa M, Sugarbaker DJ: Benign schwannoma of the esophagus presenting as a giant fibrovascular polyp. *Ann Thorac Surg* 1992; **53:** 343–345

50. Prevot S, Bienvenu L, Vaillant JC, de Saint-Maur PP: Benign schwannoma of the digestive tract. A clinicopathological and immunohistochemical study of five cases including a case of esophageal tumor. *Am J Surg Pathol* 1999; **23:** 431–436

Polyps of the Stomach

NY Haboubi

INTRODUCTION

Gastric polyps are amongst the commonest in the gastrointestinal tract. It has been estimated that they are found in 2–3% of all gastric endoscopic examinations.[1] They have, however, unfortunately suffered an abuse of terminology which has led to confusion. For instance in some series fundic glandular cystic polyps are by far the commonest polyps found and yet there is no reference to this polyp type in other large series.[1]

To add to the complexity, the gastric mucosa (unlike the rest of the gastrointestinal tract) is a complex structure with numerous cell types that are seen in varying amounts in the different regions. In theory any or all of the special cell types in any region can proliferate and produce a polyp.

Furthermore, it is relatively more common for the biopsy of a polyp to reveal histologically normal mucosa in the stomach than it is elsewhere in the gastrointestinal tract. In our experience, it is not uncommon to receive gastric biopsies from an endoscopically apparent polyp only to reveal normal gastric mucosa. This polyp can be the result of either a submucosal tumour *or* simply due to heaped up mucosa. In two series[2,3] up to 18% of the gastric polyps had histologically normal mucosa.

NORMAL STRUCTURE

Anatomy

The stomach is divided grossly into three main parts:

- The *cardia*, which is a small, ill-defined zone between 0.5 and 3 cm from the gastro-oesophageal junction.

- The *antrum*, which is the distal third of the stomach, proximal to the pyloric sphincter.

- In North America the remainder of the stomach is referred to as the *fundus*. In Britain the fundus is regarded as consisting solely of the small portion of stomach that lies superior to the lower end of the oesophagus. The main portion of the stomach is called the *body* or the *corpus*. In this chapter we will use the British topographical terminology.

These regions are not fixed anatomical zones. They merge with each other and vary according to the individual and age.[4]

Histologically, the gastric mucosa consists of three zones, which correspond roughly, but not precisely, to the gross anatomical regions. From the lower oesophagus extending distally for approximately 0.5–3 cm is the cardiac mucosa where the gastric glands are mucus-secreting. Extending from the pylorus proximally is the pyloric mucosa where the glands are also mucus-secreting. This zone is triangular, extending much further along the lesser than the greater curvature.[4] Usually the pyloric mucosa extends for 3–4 cm proximally from the pylorus along the greater curvature and from 5 cm proximal to the pylorus as far, even, as the cardia along the lesser curvature. The pathologist and endoscopist should note that the pyloric mucosal zone is *not* identical with the gross anatomy of the antrum, although some authors use these terms interchangeably. When the pathologist receives a specimen designated by the endoscopist as 'body or fundus' and finds only antral type mucosa, there should be no pathological conclusions in the report. Elsewhere within the stomach the mucosa is exclusively of the fundic type. There the glands are specialised for the secretion of acid, pepsin, intrinsic factor and blood group substances. Histological transition between the zones is gradual and junctional mucosa, which is commonly up to 1 cm in width, will show mixed features.

Histology

The surface is lined by tall columnar mucus-secreting cells and is similar throughout the mucosal zones of the stomach. The surface invaginates into the subjacent tissue to form pits, crypts or foveolae, which are lined by surface epithelial cells (Fig 2.1). The mucus in these cells is neutral, periodic acid-Schiff (PAS) positive and Alcian Blue negative at pH 2.5 and 1, respectively.

Cardiac and antral zones

In these zones, the foveolae occupy approximately one-half of the thickness of the mucosa. The subjacent glands are coiled and occasionally branched. They are exclusively mucus-secreting and are loosely packed together with abundant intervening lamina propria (Fig 2.2). The packing of the glands is slightly looser in the cardia than in the pylorus.

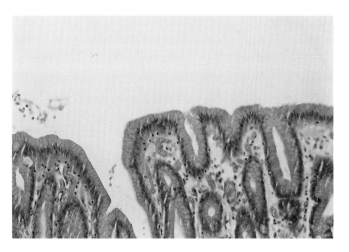

Figure 2.1 – This shows gastric surface epithelial cells dipping into the fovcolar pits.

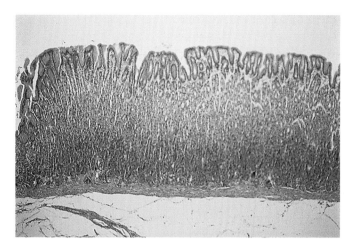

Figure 2.3 – This shows body type gastric mucosa where the crypts are straight and are composed mostly of specialised cells. This type occupies most of the mucosa.

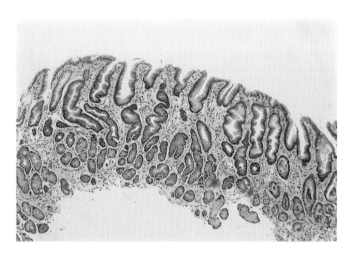

Figure 2.2 – This photomicrograph is from the pyloric region where the glands are essentially made up of mucus-secreting cells.

Body mucosa

The mucosa of the body of the stomach has pits that are shorter than elsewhere, occupying only one-quarter of the thickness of the mucosa. In contrast to the cardiac and pyloric mucosa, the glands are straight (Fig 2.3) and are divided into three zones: the base, neck and isthmus. The basal part of the gland consists mainly of chief (pepsin-secreting) cells. These have a basally situated nucleus and their cytoplasm usually stains a pale grey-blue with haematoxylin and eosin (H&E). The isthmic portion of the gland contains predominantly parietal (acid-secreting) cells. These

are roughly triangular with their bases along the basement membrane. The nuclei are centrally placed and the cytoplasm stains deep pink with H&E. In addition to acid secretion, these cells also secrete intrinsic factor and blood group substances. The neck portion of the gland contains a mixture of chief and parietal cells together with a third type, the mucus neck cell which contains a similar type of mucin to that of the surface epithelium. The mucus neck cells (located in the neck and isthmic portions of the glands from all areas of the stomach) have the functional capability of proliferating and hence regenerating the mucosa, i.e. they act as stem cells which migrate 'upwards' to renew the mucus-secreting surface epithelium or 'downwards' to form chief, parietal and neuroendocrine cells. Small proportions of neuroendocrine cells are seen in the mucosa. They form a heterogeneous population that includes enterochromaffin, enterochromaffin-like (ECL), D, Gx, X_1, D_1 and P cells.[5] Most of these cells are argyrophilic.[6] Most of the G-cells are seen in the antro–pyloric mucosa and the majority of ECL-cells are in the body.

Gastric rugae

These are numerous longitudinal, greyish pink mucosal folds, which characterise the gastric body. They lie parallel to the lesser curvature and are most prominent in the greater curve and fundus because it is this area that dilates to accommodate food. Their appearance is more prominent when the stomach is empty; they disappear completely when the stomach is dilated (Fenoglio-Preiser *et al*: pp. 137).[7]

PANCREATIC HETEROTOPIAS

Synonyms

Heterotopic pancreatic tissue, heterotopic pancreas.

Prevalence

This is the commonest gastric heterotopia (Fenoglio-Preiser *et al*: pp. 156).[7]

Endoscopic appearance

- Pancreatic heterotopia usually appears as a solitary submucosal, hemispheric, umbilicated mass measuring up to 4 cm in diameter.

- Sometimes it can be multiple and polypoidal.

- It is mostly seen in the antrum, followed by the pylorus and the greater curvature.

Microscopic features

Most of the lesions lie in the submucosa.

They are composed of normal pancreatic acini, ducts, islets and often hypertrophied muscle fibres (Fig 2.5).

They are sometimes associated with other gastric or Brunner gland heterotopias.

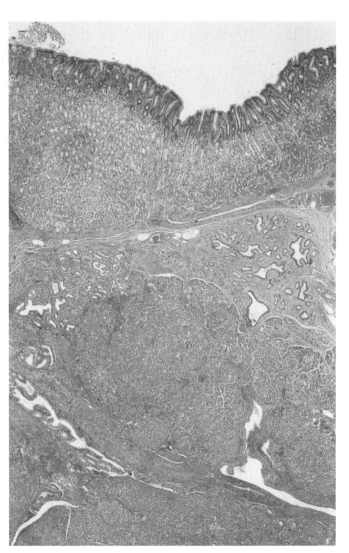

Figure 2.5 – This is a photomicrograph of a pancreatic heterotopia showing normal gastric surface epithelium and the presence of a pancreatic ducts and acini in the submucosa.

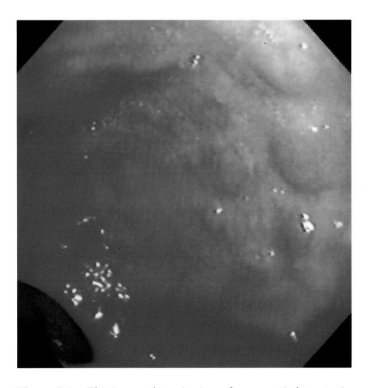

Figure 2.4 – This is an endoscopic view of a pancreatic heterotopia, which appears as a submucosal elevation with smooth covering mucosa.

Biological behaviour and associated conditions

They are mostly asymptomatic and discovered incidentally during endoscopy.

Occasionally they can be complicated by inflammation, cyst formation or neoplasia.

Management

No treatment is required if asymptomatic.

GASTRIC GLAND HETEROTOPIA

Synonyms

Gastric heterotopia, gastritis cystica profunda.

Prevalence

This is found in 0.5–11% of resected stomachs and in 1–13.7% of autopsies.[8]

Mostly seen in the seventh decade of life (Fenoglio-Preiser *et al*: p. 156).[7]

Endoscopic appearance

- Bulging lesion in the submucosa or the muscularis of the body and/or antrum.

Microscopic features

In the more common forms, there is displacement of the gastric epithelium into the submucosa (Fig 2.6). The surface immediately overlying the lesion may appear to be atrophic and may show evidence of chronic gastritis.

Biological behaviour and associated conditions

Usually associated with chronic gastritis and has no malignant predisposition.

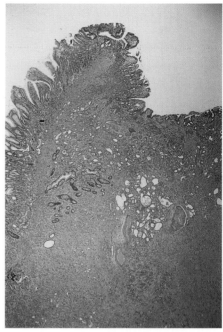

A

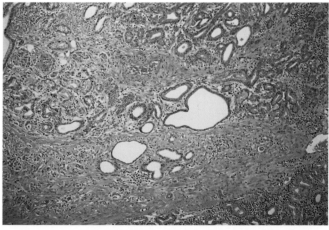

B

Figure 2.6 – (*a*) This shows an antral-type gastric mucosa with submucosal extension of the benign glandular tissue making the complex of gastritis cystica profunda. (*b*) A higher power view showing the herniation of the antral-type glands into the submucosa.

Management

Conservative.

JUVENILE POLYPS

Synonyms

Hamartoma.

Prevalence

Gastric polyps are frequently part of the syndrome of juvenile polyposis. Occasionally, they can be found as solitary polyps in the stomach.[9] (See also p. 131 in Chapter 6).

In the syndrome of gastric juvenile polyposis, the multiple polyps are predominantly found in the stomach at the initial presentation. Indeed, the stomach may remain as the only site of these lesions, although usually other polyps are seen in the small and large intestine.[10]

Endoscopic appearance

- If associated with generalised polyposis, the polyps may cover most of the mucosa (Fig 2.7).

- They can be complicated by erosions and secondary infection.[11]

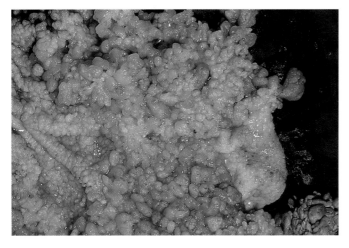

Figure 2.7 – Surgical specimen of a case of familial gastric juvenile polyposis. Note the variable size of the polyps which cover the entire specimen.

Microscopic features

Gastric juvenile polyps may resemble hyperplastic polyps or polyps associated with Cronkhite–Canada syndrome. It is therefore important to remember that a definitive diagnosis requires the full knowledge of the clinical features such as age, symptoms, distribution and number of polyps.

The polyps are characterised by:

- Irregular hyperplasia and cystic change of the foveolae (Figs 2.8–2.10). Sometimes Paneth cells may be prominent.

- Initially normal, but later atrophic, gastric specialised cells.

- Separation of polyps by oedematous superficial lamina propria.

- Variable degree of mixed inflammatory cell infiltrate in the glands and the surrounding tissue.

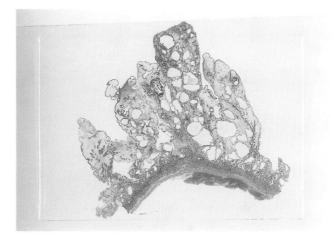

Figure 2.8 – A whole tissue mount of a juvenile polyp. Note the cystic dilatation.

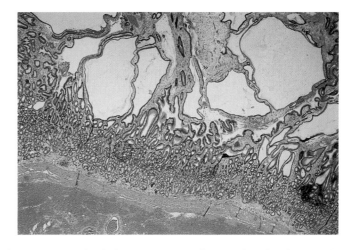

Figure 2.9 – This higher power view of a juvenile polyp shows oedematous and inflamed stroma investing dilated cystic crypts.

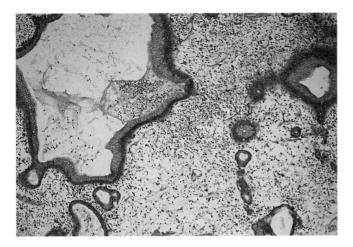

Figure 2.10 – A higher power view of the lining epithelium of the dilated glands.

Biological behaviour and associated conditions

Sometimes there are surface erosions with bleeding and outlet obstruction. Such complications may warrant gastrectomy.

Individual polyps may develop carcinomatous changes.

The syndrome of juvenile polyposis is associated with a high incidence of gastrointestinal malignancy, not necessarily in the stomach and surveillance is necessary.[9,12]

Neoplastic transformation in gastric juvenile polyposis occurs in 25% of cases.[10]

Management

Patients with single juvenile polyps are treated conservatively.

Patients with juvenile polyps containing dysplasia should be in a clinical follow-up programme that facilitates the early detection of carcinoma (Fenoglio-Preiser *et al*: p. 739).[7]

PEUTZ–JEGHERS POLYPS

Synonyms

Hamartomatous polyps.

Prevalence

Polyps are found in the stomach in 24% of cases (Ming: p. 139)[13] of Peutz–Jeghers syndrome.

The incidence is equal for both sexes.[14]

They are almost always associated with intestinal polyposis although they occasionally appear as isolated gastric polyps.[15]

Endoscopic appearance

- They are usually multiple and vary in size and shape (Fig 2.11).

- They can be sessile or pedunculated.

- The larger polyps are made up of lobules, each lobule having the typical histological features of a small Peutz–Jeghers polyp.

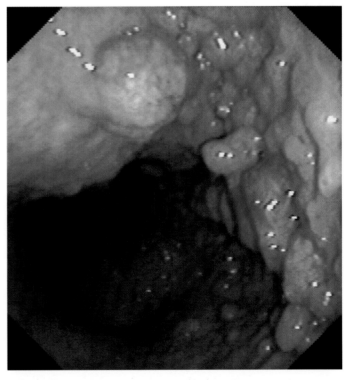

Figure 2.11 – An endoscopic view of a case of Peutz–Jeghers polyps showing multiple polyps of various sizes in the stomach.

Microscopic features

In the stomach the polyps are different from those found in the colon and small intestine, where there is a more balanced proliferation of epithelial and stromal components (Watanabe *et al*: p. 35).[11]

The gastric polyps show: hyperplastic mucus cells, elongation and cystic changes of foveolar epithelium, reduced lamina propria and prominent branching bands of muscularis mucosae derived from smooth muscle (Fig 2.12).

Submucosal misplacement of glands is common and should not be interpreted as a malignant change.

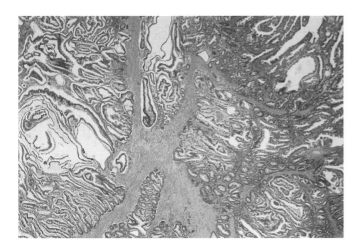

Figure 2.12 – A photomicrographic view of Peutz–Jeghers polyp. There are branching complexes of hyperplastic mucous cells and prominent muscle fibres, which are very characteristic of these polyps.

Biological behaviour and associated conditions

(See p. 134 in Chapter 6). The full clinical picture of Peutz–Jeghers polyps is characterised by:

- Gastrointestinal polyposis.
- Oral pigmentation.
- Autosomal dominant inheritance.

Formes frustes are sometimes seen where, for example, the oral pigmentation is absent.

Malignant changes in the polyps are rare but have been recorded in gastric Peutz–Jeghers polyps.[16] The development of tumours outside the stomach, or even outside the gastrointestinal tract (such as in the ovary, cervix, testis, pancreas and breast) is well described.[17]

Management

The treatment of choice is polypectomy and surveillance.

CRONKHITE–CANADA POLYPS

Synonyms

Hamartoma.

Prevalence

Multiple gastric polyps are seen in almost all cases of Cronkhite–Canada syndrome (CCS), which is characterised (in addition to gastrointestinal polyposis) by protein-losing enteropathy, alopecia, nail atrophy and skin pigmentation.[18] (See also p. 138 in Chapter 6).

Endoscopic appearance

- Multiple polyps ranging from pinhead to cherry size (Watanabe *et al*: p. 37)[11] with frequent superficial erosions.
- The polyp-bearing mucosa is noticeably thickened and may be ulcerated.
- There are close similarities between the gastric changes in CCS and Menetrier's disease.

Microscopic features

The polyps are characterised by:

- Intact mucosa as a rule, ulceration being uncommon.
- Proliferation of tortuous glands (some filled with inspissated proteinaceous material or mucus).
- The mucosa between the polyps shows oedema, congestion inflammation and focal glandular ectasia (Fig 2.13).
- The polyps of juvenile polyposis are often indistinguishable from those of CCS, but they differ from CCS in that the intervening mucosa is histologically normal.[18]

Biological behaviour and associated conditions

The polyps may grow in size and may sometimes regress, usually with treatment.

There is a low malignant potential.

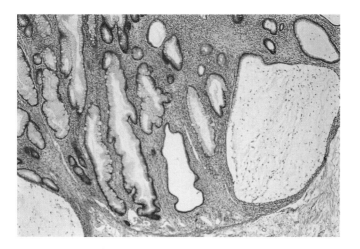

Figure 2.13 – A case of Cronkhite–Canada syndrome in which inflamed and oedematous stroma surround dilated glands lined by simple mucous secreting cells. Note the similarity to juvenile polyp.

Management

No specific treatment is required for the individual polyp. Intense supportive medical therapy, including nutritional support, is usually required. Resection of severely affected bowel segments may relieve the protein loss.

HYPERPLASTIC POLYPS

Synonyms

Hyperplasiogenous polyps, regenerative polyps, hyperplastic adenomatous polyps, Nakamura types I and II polyps, inflammatory polyps.

Prevalence

In most series these are the commonest gastric polyps.

They are also the commonest polyps seen in the gastric stump or at a gastric anastomotic site. They are also seen at the site of, or bordering, an ulcer or erosion.[19]

In one study of stomachs operated upon for benign gastric ulcers,[20] hyperplastic polyps were found in 12.1% of Billroth II resections and in 14.9% of gasteroenterostomies, mostly close to the gasteroenterostomy.

Endoscopic appearance

- They vary from a few millimetres to 4 cm in diameter and are usually, but not always, in the antrum (Fig 2.14).

- They are usually multiple (Fig 2.15).

- When small, they have a smooth, dome-shaped appearance, often with a depression in the centre.

- They sometimes take the shape of bulbous projections on the surface of the gastric folds.

- Larger lesions may appear to be lobulated and to have a stalk.

- They feel spongy in consistency.

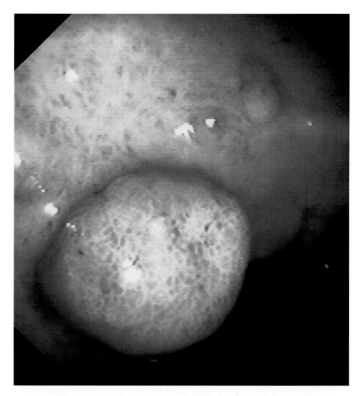

Figure 2.14 – Endoscopic view of a regenerative/hyperplastic polyp. This view shows a single polypoidal lesion in the gastric antrum.

Microscopic features

The microscopic features[21] are characterised by:

- Elongated and tortuous foveolae that are lined by mucus-secreting cells (Figs 2.16 & 2.17).

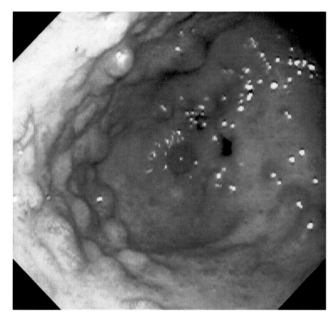

Figure 2.15 – In this case multiple regenerative/hyperplastic polyps are seen in the antrum.

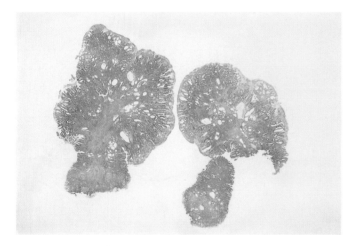

Figure 2.16 – This shows a whole tissue mount of a regenerative hyperplastic polyp, divided in two, showing cystic dilatation in the prominent stroma.

- The presence of normal antral, or less commonly body-type, glands in the deeper part of the polyp.

- In the lamina propria there is oedema, a variable degree of mixed inflammatory cell infiltration and smooth muscle fibres originating from the muscularis mucosae.

- In approximately 10% of cases there is intestinal metaplasia.

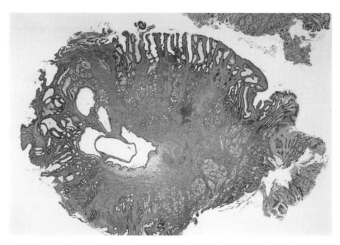

Figure 2.17 – This is a higher power view of a regenerative/hyperplastic polyp in which there is foveolar hyperplasia and cystic dilatation of the antral-type glandular tissue invested in a fibrotic stroma containing chronic inflammatory cell infiltrate.

- In cases of surface ulceration, the regenerating cells are cuboidal with eosinophilic cytoplasm and a large central nucleus ('Pinky cells').[21]

These features are usually identified in a completely resected polyp or gastrectomy resectate, but may be difficult to find in a biopsy. Consequently, multiple levels *may* be needed.

Biological behaviour and associated conditions

They are mostly innocuous and found in a background of chronic gastritis.

Carcinoma has reportedly arisen in solitary hyperplastic polyps in 0.3–1% of cases.[22] Nevertheless, the incidence of synchronous or metachronous gastric carcinoma range from 1.2–2.8%. This indicates that these polyps have a low malignant potential although they may act as a marker for a neoplastic process elsewhere in the stomach.

In 8% of cases hyperplastic polyps are multiple. In these circumstances, carcinoma has been reported in up to 36% of the polyps and synchronous carcinoma has been reported in up to 57% of cases.

A possible association with *Helicobacter pylori* has been reported.[23]

Sometimes, there is a combination of dysplastic epithelium with non-neoplastic epithelium.

Management

For solitary polyps excision is adequate. For multiple polyps regular follow-up is recommended.[24] They often recur after polypectomy.[25]

FOCAL FOVEOLAR HYPERPLASIAS

Synonyms

Pit hyperplasias, polypoid foveolar hyperplasias, foveolar hyperplasias, focal foveolar glandular hyperplasias.

Prevalence

Different authors have different opinions. In one series from Germany this condition accounted for 92% of mucosal polyps[26] whereas another series from Finland suggested that this polyp accounted for only 20% of gastric polyps.[27]

Endoscopic appearance

- They are small, sessile elevations and may measure up to 5 mm in diameter (Fig 2.18).

- They occur in the antrum or body and are usually multiple.[28]

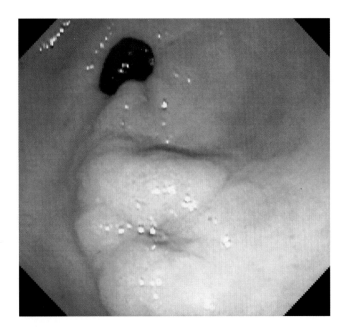

Figure 2.18 – An endoscopic view of a case of focal foveolar hyperplasia.

Microscopic features

Elongation of the foveolar portion of the mucosa without any alteration of the underlying glandular elements (Fig 2.19).

Normal or slightly hyperchromatic foveolar cells.

There may be surface erosion with accompanying degenerative or regenerative changes.

Occasionally, there is intestinal metaplasia.

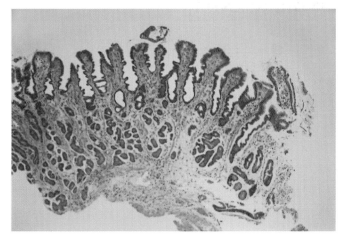

A

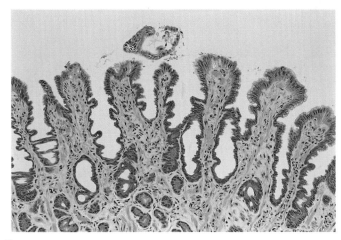

B

Figure 2.19 – (*a*) A photomicrograph of a case of focal foveolar hyperplasia. Some workers consider them as early forms of hyperplastic polyps. These lesions are characterised by an elongation of foveolar cells with or without surface erosions. (*b*) A high power view showing the hyperplastic foveolar cells covering the papillary configuration of the polyp.

Biological behaviour and associated conditions

These are common polypoidal lesions, which are seen in association with duodenal and gastric ulcers, gastric carcinoma and gastrojejunostomy with other polyps.[28]

They have been regarded by some workers[28] as an early or incipient stage of hyperplastic polyps.

These polyps are benign and there is no increased risk of carcinoma.[29]

Management

Polypectomy is adequate treatment.

FUNDIC GLAND POLYPS

Synonyms

Fundic gland cyst polyps, fundic gland hyperplasias, fundic gland polyposis, cystic hamartomatous gastric polyps, cysts of the glandular body, Elster's cysts, polyps with fundic glandular cyst.

Prevalence

These polyps are seen more commonly in women with a ratio of 5:1.[30]

They constitute the commonest type of gastric polyps in some, but not all series.[31] This may be due to differences in terminology.

They are the commonest type of gastric polyps in patients with familial adenomatous polyposis (FAP).[32] Roughly 30–50% of FAP patients have these polyps and they are usually demonstrated in the second and third decade of life.

In the general population however, they are acquired in middle age.[33]

Endoscopic appearance

- Sometimes single but usually multiple (Fig 2.20), 1–5 mm in diameter, restricted to the body and fundus (i.e. the acid-secreting zone).

- They are small, mostly sessile, dome-shaped lesions with a glassy transparent appearance.

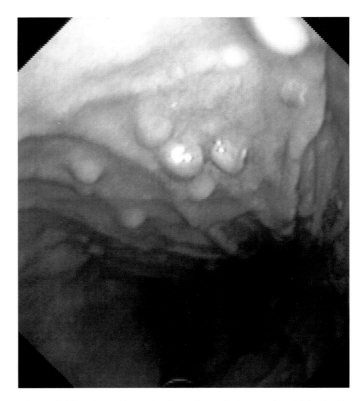

Figure 2.20 – An endoscopic view of a typical case of multiple fundic cystic gland polyps. Sometimes the lesion can be solitary.

Microscopic features

Fundic gland polyps are characterised by:

- Their location in the body-type mucosa.

- Scattered cysts lined by foveolar and body glandular epithelium (including parietal and chief cells) (Figs 2.21 & 2.22).

- Body-type gastric acinar hyperplasia near the surface.

- Short pits (sometimes).

- Normal lamina propria.

- In exceptionally rare circumstances, focal dysplasia.

Biological behaviour and associated conditions

Initially reported in association with FAP. Subsequently, it has been found that they also occur in patients without FAP.

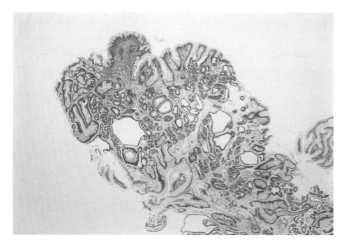

Figure 2.21 – A low power photomicrograph of a fundic gland polyp showing dilated cystic structures.

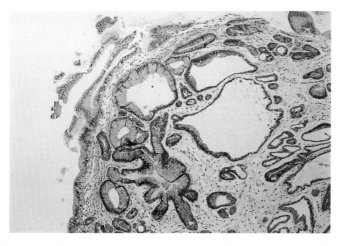

Figure 2.22 – A higher power view of a fundic gland polyp showing that the cysts are lined in parts by fovoelar and in parts by specialised gastric cells.

Spontaneous regression may take place in patients with[34] or without FAP.[33] However, in patients with FAP the tendency is to increase in size *and* number (see p. 126 in Chapter 6).

Some reports suggest a strong association with long-term omeprazole intake.[35]

A rare syndrome, which is associated with multiple fundic glandular polyps and cutaneous psoriasis, has been reported and may represent a syndrome with an autosomal dominant mode of inheritance (Fenoglio-Preiser *et al*: p. 740).[7]

Management

They are neither precancerous nor do they require prophylactic surgery.

When hundreds of these polyps are present there is a strong indication of FAP (Watanabe *et al*: p. 35)[11] and therefore colonoscopy is advisable.

ANTRAL GLAND HYPERPLASIA

Synonyms

Brunner's gland adenoma, heterotopic adenomatous polyp.

Prevalence

Very rare lesion.

Endoscopic appearance

- This appears as a nipple-like projection above the mucosal surface (Ming: p. 141)[13] of the antrum.

Microscopic features

This polyp is characterised by:

- Proliferation of antral glands in clusters separated by bundles of smooth muscles.[21]
- Normal foveolae.[21]
- Sparse, or absent, inflammation.[21]

Biological behaviour and associated conditions

Benign and not known to be associated with other systemic or localised pathology.

HYPERTROPHIED GASTROPATHIES

When the gastric mucosa is thickened and measures more than 1.5 mm in depth, this may be the result of a process of hyperplasia or hypertrophy (Fenoglio-Preiser *et al*: p. 209).[7] The local or diffuse mucosal expansions result in giant mucosal folds (hypertrophic gastropathy) producing characteristic gross, endoscopic and radiological appearances. The hypertrophy may affect either or both mucosal components i.e. the superficial epithelium with foveolar cells and/or the subjacent specialised cells.

There are at least two well defined variants of hypertrophic gastropathy:

- Menetrier's disease.

- Hypersecretory hypergastrinaemia, with protein loss (Zollinger–Ellison syndrome).

MENETRIER'S DISEASE

Synonyms

Gastric hypertrophy with protein loss and hypochlorhydria.

Prevalence

There are two types: the adult form, which is seen mostly in men in their sixth decade of life[28] and a second type which is very rare and is seen in children and young infants, where it is usually a self-limiting disease.

Endoscopic/gross appearance

- Thickened and marked enlargement of the gastric mucosal folds (Fig 2.23), which can be localised or diffuse.

- The folds vary from 1–3 cm in height and in many ways resemble cerebral convolutions.

- In the adult form, the disease affects the body and greater curvatures sparing the antrum.

- In children however, the antrum is more greatly affected.

Microscopic features

There is foveolar hyperplasia lining tortuous, dilated hyperplastic gastric pits (Fig 2.24).

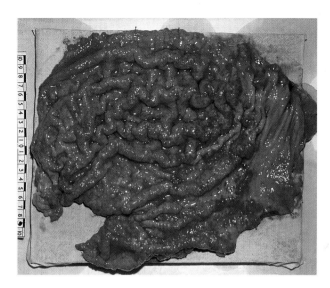

Figure 2.23 – Gross appearance of a case of hypertrophied gastropathy (Menetrier's disease) showing exaggerated folds throughout the specimen. Note the similarity to cerebral convolutions.

There is atrophy of the specialised glandular components. Sometimes there is cystic dilatation at the end of the pit.

There is a variable degree of inflammation and superficial oedema.

Sometimes the elongated and dilated pits extend into the submucosa to produce gastritis cytica profunda.

Hyperplasia and hypertrophy of the muscularis mucosae occurs as a secondary phenomenon.

It is important to note that some, or all, of the above histological features can be seen in other conditions such as prolapsed gastrostomy mucosa, reflux gastropathy, at the margins of peptic ulcers and even in hyperplastic polyps. It is therefore *imperative*, when considering the diagnosis of Menetrier's disease, to take into account the clinical and endoscopic features.

Biological behaviour and associated conditions

In the adult population there is usually epigastric pain, bloating, anorexia, vomiting, weight loss and peripheral oedema. There is protein loss, hypoalbuminaemia and hypochlorhydria. In over 60% of patients there is an associated eosinophilia.

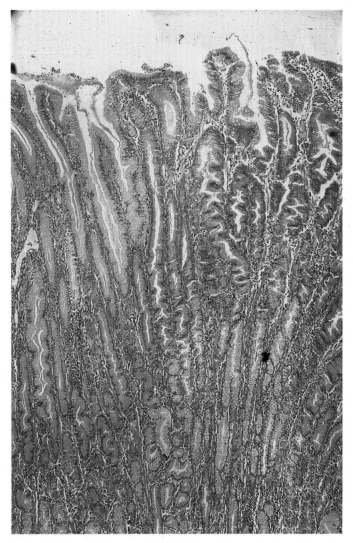

Figure 2.24 – A histological section of a case of Menetrier's disease showing the hyperplastic gastric pits and atrophy of the specialised gastric epithelium.

The extra-intestinal manifestations include recurrent pulmonary infection, pulmonary oedema and thrombotic cardiovascular disease.

There are reports that suggest that gastric carcinoma coexists with Menetrier's disease but this association is not clear.

As the disease advances, the degree of hypochlorhydria progresses. This is due to the replacement of the acid-secreting cells with foveolar cells.

In the paediatric population the disease is very rare and is usually self-limiting. There is an association with allergy, autoimmune reaction and cytomegalovirus infection.[36] There is usually oedema, abdominal pain and anorexia.

MUCOSAL FOLD HYPERTROPHY ASSOCIATED WITH ZOLLINGER–ELLISON SYNDROME

Prevalence

The Zollinger–Ellison syndrome affects 0.1% of patients with duodenal ulcers.

There is no major sex predominance.

The condition is estimated to affect 0.2–0.4 patients/million population per year.

There is a wide range (from 7–90 years) in age incidence. Most patients are diagnosed in the third to fifth decades of life.

Endoscopic appearance

- The giant folds characteristically cover the body and fundus and spare the antrum.

Microscopic features

There is substantial glandular lengthening due to an increased number of parietal cells. The increased parietal cell mass forms the larger share of the glands and may fill their entire length down to their base.

The foveolae may be normal in length or shortened.

Biological behaviour and associated conditions

The commonest presenting symptoms are abdominal pain, steatorrhoea and peptic ulceration.

Not all symptoms are necessarily present at the time of presentation.

GASTRIC XANTHELASMA

Synonyms

Xanthoma, lipid islands.

Prevalence

These lesions have been noted endoscopically in 0.4–6.3% of non-operated patients[37,38] but are more prevalent in patients with gastric stumps particularly those of substantial duration. It has been reported that 60% of patients who have had Billroth II operations have these lesions after 20 years or more of follow-up.[37]

Endoscopic appearance

- Mostly single, sometimes multiple, well demarcated, circular or oval, whitish-yellow lesions measuring 1–2 mm in diameter (rarely exceeding 5 mm in diameter).

Microscopic features

They consist entirely (or sometimes mainly) of lipid containing histiocytes (xanthoma cells) arranged in pavement-like sheets in the upper lamina propria, immediately beneath the surface epithelium. They can be intermingled with lymphocytes, plasma cells, macrophages and other mononuclear cells.

Biological behaviour and associated conditions

Usually associated with pathology in the stomach especially chronic gastritis and peptic ulcer disease.

Management

No surgical management or follow-up is required.

INFLAMMATORY FIBROID POLYP

Synonyms

Eosinophilic granuloma, granuloblastoma, xanthofibroma, eosinophilic pseudotumour, haemangioendothelioma, haemangiopericytoma, Vanek polyp.

Prevalence

Inflammatory fibroid polyp (IFP) is a rare condition, which can occur anywhere in the gastrointestinal tract. The stomach is the most frequently affected organ.[39]

In one large series, IFP accounted for 4.5% of all gastric polyps.[40] This may not be a true reflection of the incidence, since foveolar hyperplasia and polypoid regenerative elevations were excluded in that particular series.

Female to male ratio is 1.6:1, with a wide age incidence peaking between the 5th and 8th decades of life.

Endoscopic appearance

- Mostly solitary, partly submucosal and partly mucosal lesions ranging between 0.5 and 1.5 cm (occasionally over 2 cm) in diameter.

- The majority are located in the antrum. Other parts of the stomach are rarely involved.

- Surface erosion or ulceration can be seen in up to 30% of cases.

Microscopic features

The basic component is a proliferation of fibroblasts and blood vessels infiltrated by a variable number of eosinophils (Watanabe et al: p. 37),[11] and, to a lesser extent, neutrophils and plasma cells (Figs 2.25 & 2.26).

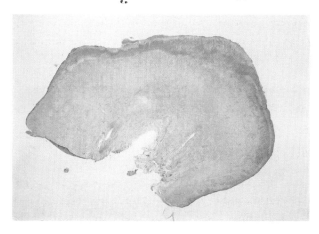

Figure 2.25 – A low power view of an inflammatory fibroid polyp showing dense stroma with attenuated lining epithelium.

Figure 2.26 – A higher power view showing the fibrovascular proliferation that characterises these IFP lesions.

The fibroblastic proliferation has a characteristic onion skin orientation around small blood vessels.

In the majority of cases, there is a significant loss of the muscularis mucosae.

Approximately 50% of the lesions involve the mucosa only, with 45% involving the mucosa and submucosa. It is rare to see the lesion involving the submucosa only.

Immunohistochemically, there may be either myofibroblastic or histiocytic lines of differentiation, indicating a heterogeneity that may reflect the stage of development.[41]

Biological behaviour and associated conditions

Despite a sometimes dramatic endoscopic appearance this is purely a reactive, non-neoplastic lesion.

It does not recur after polypectomy and is not known to be associated with other conditions.

Management

These lesions often come to polypectomy or even local surgery because they are not diagnosed adequately by biopsy. Once the diagnosis is made, no further resection or surveillance is required because these are benign non-neoplastic lesions.

ADENOMA

Synonyms

Papillary adenoma, villous adenoma, adenomatous dysplasia.

Prevalence

It is difficult to obtain an accurate assessment of prevalence. In one paper,[22] which excluded fundic cystic gland polyps, mesenchymal tumours and polypoidal lymphomas, adenomas constituted 19.6% of the remainder of the gastric polyps studied.

Endoscopic appearance

- They usually appear as soft, sessile or broad based lesions (Figs 2.27 & 2.28).

- Adenomas are mostly seen in the antrum and are usually larger than 2 cm in diameter (Ming: p. 71).[13]

- Red discolouration and surface ulceration are suggestive endoscopic signs of malignant transformation (Ming: p. 71).[13,21]

Microscopic features

Circumscribed neoplasm composed of tubular and/or villous structures lined by dysplastic epithelium. There are three histological types (Watanabe *et al*: pp. 19–20).[11]

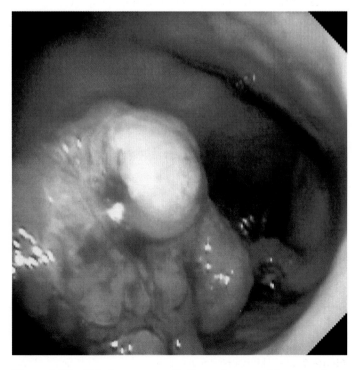

Figure 2.27 – This shows a case of solitary adenoma of the stomach.

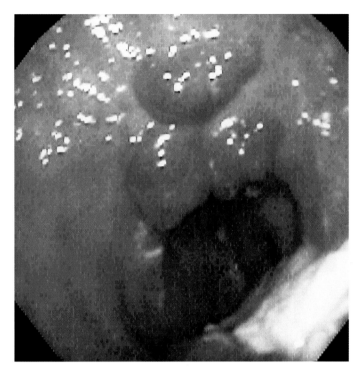

Figure 2.28 – This shows a rare case of multiple gastric adenomas.

- *Tubular.* This is composed of tubules surrounded by lamina propria.

- *Villous (papillary).* This is composed of finger-like neoplastic cells with a core of lamina propria.

- *Tubulovillous (papillotubular).* This is composed of both tubular and villous structures, each contributing at least 20% to the tumour (Fig 2.29).

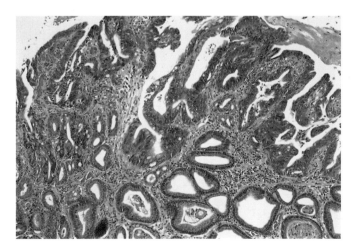

Figure 2.29 – This is a photomicrograph of a case of gastric tubulovillous adenoma.

Gastric adenomas share the histological classification applied to colonic adenomas but differ from the latter in the following points:

- Gastric adenomas are much less common.

- Most gastric tubular adenomas are slightly raised or sessile rather than pedunculated lesions. As in the colon, adenomas can be flat or even depressed, i.e. non-polypoidal.

Classically in gastric adenomas, the dysplastic epithelium occupies the upper part of the polyp while the subjacent portion of the adenoma can remain non-neoplastic; either with some cystic change or remaining completely normal (Watanabe *et al*: pp. 19–20).[11]

Tubular adenomas are more common than villous or tubulovillous. However the latter two patterns are more common in carcinoma than in adenoma of the stomach.

Biological behaviour and associated conditions

Malignant transformation is related to the size, and is rarely seen (less than 2% of cases) with adenomas that are under 2 cm in diameter. However, malignancy has been found in 40–50% of adenomas that are larger than 2 cm (Ming: p. 71).[13] It has been estimated that about 5% of early gastric cancers arise in adenomas.[42]

Management

Polypectomy is the treatment of choice.

Because there is a risk of developing metachronous neoplasia, post-polypectomy endoscopic/biopsy follow-up is recommended (Ming: p. 71).[13]

POLYPOIDAL CARCINOMA

Synonyms

Bormann's type I polyp, Nakamura type 3 polyp, carcinomatous polyp.

Prevalence

This is a relatively uncommon form of gastric cancer. It accounts for up to 8% of gastric carcinomas.

Endoscopic appearance

- Typically these lesions mimic villous adenomas (Ming: p. 164).[13] They form a sharply delineated luminal mass (Fig 2.30).

- Some secrete excessive mucus, which may produce a gelatinous or colloidal appearance.

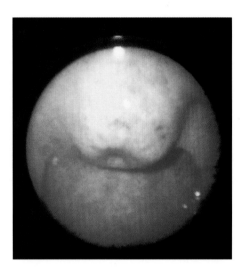

Figure 2.30 – This shows an endoscopic view of a case of polypoidal carcinoma.

Microscopic features

Usually seen as a mucus-secreting adenocarcinoma with a variable degree of papillary or signet ring formation.

The neoplasm may or may not involve the entire wall, although usually the submucosal spread is limited.

Biological behaviour and associated conditions

These tumours are, in the opinion of some workers, malignant from their inception and are therefore biologically different from carcinomas that arise in benign polyps.[43] Nevertheless, they have a limited invasive potential (Ming: p. 164).[13]

Management

Whilst total polypectomy may result in cure, many advocate a limited gastrectomy for these lesions.[23,44] After the initial forceps biopsy, if there is a malignant element, then endoscopic polypectomy or local surgical excision is the recommended procedure. Subsequently, if the histological examination shows well or moderately differentiated carcinoma and if the neoplasm is confined to the mucosa and is completely excised, no further surgery is necessary. Surgery is indicated if the neoplasm is poorly differentiated, of signet ring appearance or if it extends into the submucosa.[23] These recommendations have been challenged[45] because lymph node metastasis is seen in 1–3% of intramucosal gastric carcinomas. Age, the patient's operative risk and the location of the polyp are all important considerations in the decision to offer excisional surgery.

POLYPOID VARIANT OF EARLY GASTRIC CARCINOMA

Synonyms

Type 1 early gastric cancer, early gastric cancer protruded type.

Prevalence

Early gastric cancer is defined as 'cancer that remains limited to the mucosa or the mucosa and submucosa regardless of the presence or absence of lymph node metastasis'.

In high incidence countries such as Japan, with the help of improved diagnostic methodologies, the incidence of early gastric cancers in resected specimens for carcinoma ranges from 30–50%.[46] In the Western world however, the incidence is probably up to 16%.[47]

Endoscopic appearance

- Slightly elevated sessile nodule ranging from a few millimetres to 2 cm or more in diameter.

- Sometimes the nodules have irregular edges.

- They occasionally arise in a background of adenomas.

Microscopic features

This type of early gastric cancer is usually a well differentiated, tubular or papillary carcinoma (Fig 2.31). Sometimes there is invasion into the submucosa (Fig 2.32).

Sometimes it is associated with a pre-existing adenoma.

Sometimes the differentiation from severe dysplasia is difficult.

In some cases immunohistochemical stains are helpful for distinguishing the sometimes scant presence of signet ring cancer cells from muciphages.

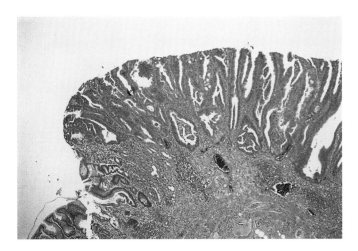

Figure 2.31 – This shows a case of the protuberant variant of early gastric cancer. The neoplasm is confined to the mucosa.

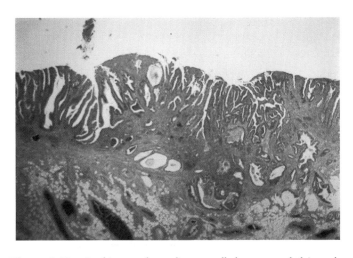

Figure 2.32 – In this case the malignant cells have extended into the submucosa but the neoplasm is still categorised as an early gastric cancer.

Biological behaviour and associated conditions

The rate of progression is very variable. In one series[48] of 56 patients, 16 did not show any progression in a mean follow-up of 29 months.

The prognosis in surgically treated gastric cancer is excellent with an expected survival rate of 95–100%.[49]

Multiple tumours carry a slightly worse prognosis.[49]

Recurrence can occasionally occur in the gastric stump after the initial surgery for early gastric cancer.

Management

Surgery is the treatment of choice.

GASTRIC CARCINOIDS

Synonyms

Neuroendocrine tumours, enterochromaffin cell-like tumours.

Prevalence

These lesions comprise less than 1% of gastric tumours.[50]

According to a range of studies, the male to female ratio is variable.

Endoscopic appearance

- They occur most frequently in the body and may be solitary or multiple small polyps (Fig 2.33).

- It is important to distinguish between the various types due to the differences in biological behaviour and the presence, or absence, of associated conditions.

Microscopic features

The neoplastic cells are regular, showing little or no pleomorphism, none or scanty mitotic figures (Fig 2.34).

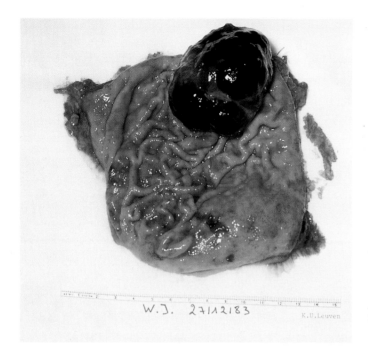

Figure 2.33 – This shows the gross appearance of a case of gastric carcinoid.

They are classically arranged in nests, trabecula or cords.

Immunohistochemically they stain positively for neuron-specific enolase, chromogranin and for a variety of polypeptides such as gastrin, 5-hydroxytryptophan, serotonin, vasoactive intestinal peptide (VIP), somatostatin and adrenocorticotrophic hormone (ACTH).

Biological behaviour and associated conditions

In view of the distinct pathological behaviour of gastric carcinoids, it has been proposed[51] that they be divided into three types:

- *Type 1.* This type is associated with type A-chronic atrophic gastritis with or without pernicious anaemia.

- *Type 2.* This type is associated with Zollinger–Ellison Syndrome (ZES) and multiple endocrine neoplasia (MEN I) (an autosomal dominant disorder characterised by tumours of the parathyroid, endocrine pancreas and anterior pituitary).

- *Type 3.* This type is sporadic.

Both Types I and 2 represent syndromes with multiple small polyps, associated with hypergastrinaemia and having a low

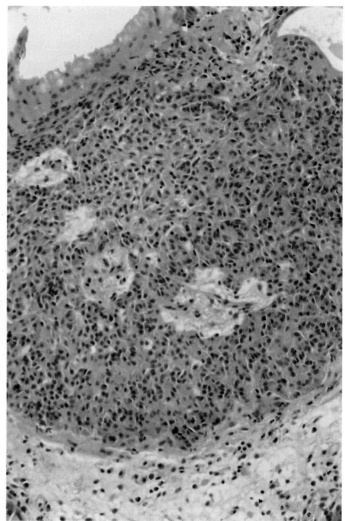

Figure 2.34 – This is a photomicrograph of a case of gastric carcinoid. Note the uniformity of the neoplastic cells that characterise these tumours.

invasive or metastasising potential (Watanabe *et al*: p. 27).[11] The neoplastic cells are predominantly enterochromaffin-like cells (ECL); hence the term ECLOMA.

It has been suggested that the gastrinaemia is a tumour promoter. In patients with pernicious anaemia or type A gastritis, it is not uncommon to see diffuse endocrine cell hyperplasia (intraglandular proliferation) and multiple endocrine cell micronests (extraglandular proliferation), followed by a progression to microcarcinoidosis.

Sporadic lesions are almost always solitary. They evolve in a background of normal gastric mucosa and display moderately aggressive behaviour with the ability to metastasise. Sometimes they can produce the carcinoid syndrome.

Gastrin levels are normal. Histologically the tumours are composed of a mixture of ECL, enterochromaffin and X-cells.

Plasma chromogranin A is elevated in all variants but more so in Type 3.[52]

Management

The recommended treatment for Types 1 and 2 is, by and large, conservative and can be divided into two phases:

- When the lesions are small or few in number (less than five), endoscopic polypectomy of the accessible lesions, followed by surveillance endoscopy at 6 monthly intervals, is recommended.[53]

- Patients with larger or more numerous lesions and patients whose tumours recur after polypectomy may be managed by antrectomy and local excision of large lesions. Antrectomy has resulted in the regression of fundic ECL in some patients, presumably due to the removal of antral G cells.

The recommended therapy for Type 3 carcinoids is en-bloc surgical resection with regional lymph node dissection.[53] In one study,[52] all patients with Type 3 carcinoid died from metastatic disease, although none of the Type 1 patients died as a result of their tumours. This study suggests that a combination therapy with interferon α and octreotide may be beneficial in patients with metastatic Type 1 gastric carcinoid disease.

GASTRIC STROMAL TUMOURS

Synonyms

Leiomyomas, leiomyosarcomas, leiomyoblastomas, smooth muscle tumours, neurilemmomas, Schwannomas, neurofibromas, gastrointestinal stromal tumours (GIST), gastrointestinal autonomic nerve tumours (GANT), stromal tumours of unknown malignant potential (STUMP).

Prevalence

Mostly affecting adults over 30 years of age with a male to female ratio of 1:1.[54]

Endoscopic appearance

- Single or multiple, varying in size from a few millimetres to over 10 cm in diameter (Fig 2.35).

- In most cases the lesions project into the lumen as exophytic polypoidal masses of various sizes and shapes (Fig 2.36).

- Large size, necrosis and/or invasion of surrounding tissue are features suggestive of malignancy.

- Although it is usually difficult to biopsy these lesions, endoscopically the benign mesenchymal submucosal tumours can be distinguished from the epithelial polyps by the following signs:

  Tent sign. The mucosa over the tumour can be raised with forceps like a tent.

  Schindler's sign. Bridging folds converging towards the tumour.

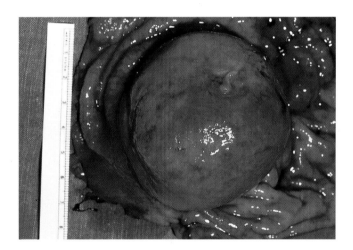

Figure 2.35 – This shows a case of benign gastric stromal tumour. Note the dome-like shape.

Microscopic features

The histogenesis of these tumours is far from being fully understood but they can be divided into four categories (as is evident from routine stains and ultrastructural features[55]):

- Tumours of smooth muscle origin.

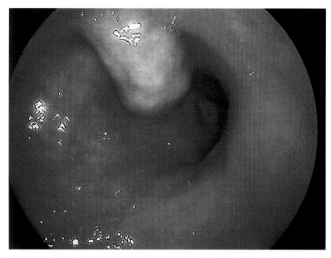

Figure 2.36 – This shows a case of a finger-like polypoidal protrusion of a benign gastric stromal tumour.

- Tumours of neural appearance but lacking the neural or neuroendocrine immunohistochemical staining.

- Tumours showing neural and smooth muscle differentiation.

- Tumours lacking any differentiation.

Recently it has been shown that the majority of stromal tumours of the stomach will express CD117 (c-kit) and CD 34 antigens, allowing these stromal tumours to be categorised by these markers as 'gastro-intestinal stromal tumours (GIST's) rather than tumours of the smooth muscle or neural origin.

All of these tumours are composed of fascicles and bundles of spindle cells, or sheets of epithelioid polygonal cells with a pink cytoplasm.

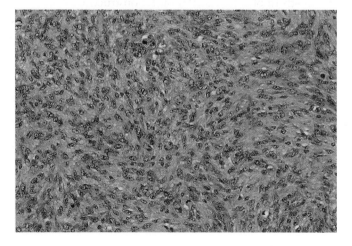

Figure 2.37 – This is a photomicrograph of a malignant gastric stromal tumour. There is dense cellularity and high mitotic count.

Features suggestive of malignancy are:

- The presence of a high mitotic count of greater than 5 in 50 high power fields (HPF) (Fig 2.37).

- Nuclear atypia.

- Intratumorous haemorrhage.

- Hypercellularity.

- Larger, or equal to, 5 cm in diameter.

- Neural differentiation.

- Necrosis.

The mucosa overlying these polyps may be entirely normal or may show features of 'compression' as shown by the shortening and slight distortion of the pits (Fig 2.38).

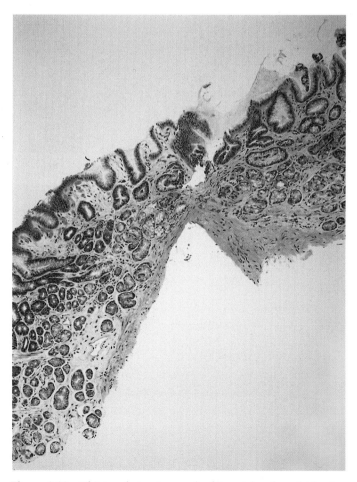

Figure 2.38 – This is a photomicrograph of tissue taken from the benign gastric stromal tumour illustrated in Fig 2.36. This figure shows the 'compressed' looking mucosa that overlies the stromal tumour.

Biological behaviour and associated conditions

Most cases are benign and are not associated with other conditions.

Occasionally the lesions can be associated with von-Recklinghausen's disease,[56] human immunodeficiency virus (HIV) infection in children and Carney syndrome (which is characterised by the triad of pulmonary chondroma, GIST and extra-adrenal paragangliomas).[57]

The most likely sites of metastasis from malignant tumours are the liver, peritoneum and lungs. These may appear up to 30 years after the removal of the primary lesion.

Management

The best treatment for malignant stromal tumours is excision with a good margin of normal tissue.[55] There is no place for simple enucleation.

Lymph node dissection is not indicated because the tumours are unlikely to metastasise to the local lymph nodes.

For benign lesions simple surgical removal is sufficient.

LIPOMA

Synonyms

Benign adipose tissue tumours.

Prevalence

This is a rare neoplasm. Most are single and located in the distal stomach.[58] The age distribution is wide.

Endoscopic appearance

- These lesions appear as lobulated, often large and soft, neoplasms arising from the submucosa (Fig 2.39).
- They may have the typical appearance for 'pillow sign', which is the impression produced by the biopsy forceps on the lesion.

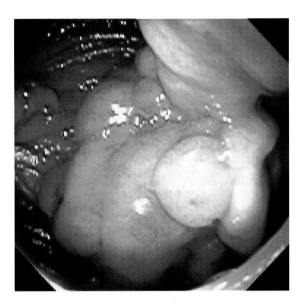

Figure 2.39 – This shows an endoscopic view of a case of gastric lipoma.

Microscopic features

They consist of lobules of mature fatty tissue separated by thin fibrovascular stroma.

Various histological changes, which are common to lipomas elsewhere, such as areas of fat necrosis, can also be found.

Biological behaviour and associated conditions

They are invariably benign. Some may bleed and give rise to iron deficiency anaemia (Ming: p. 246).[13]

In one-third of cases there is outlet obstruction.[59]

They are not known to be associated with other lesions or conditions.

Management

Polypectomy is the treatment of choice.

LYMPHOMATOUS POLYPOSIS

Synonyms

Mantle cell type malignant lymphoma, diffuse centrocytic lymphoma.

Prevalence

This is an uncommon disease, mostly seen in patients over 50 years of age[60] and usually involves a long segment of the gastrointestinal tract with predominance in the ileocaecal region (see p. 140).[61]

Gastric involvement at presentation was seen in three out of four cases reported by O'Brien et al.[62]

Endoscopic appearance

- Multiple white fleshy mucosal polyps ranging from 0.5 to 2 cm in diameter.

Microscopic features

The neoplastic cells have a centrocytic appearance, usually in a nodular background.

A characteristic feature of the neoplasm is the trapping of reactive follicles and replacement of their mantle zone.[61]

The neoplastic cells are of B-cell lineage and the immunotyping suggests derivation from a sub-population of CD5 positive mantle zone cells.[61]

Biological behaviour and associated conditions

These neoplasms have a poor prognosis and most patients will progress to extra-intestinal nodal disease. Indeed there is, more often than not, wide dissemination early in the disease to the liver, bone marrow and lymph nodes.

Management

No further surgical management or follow-up is required, specifically for the gastric disease in this syndrome.

OTHER LESIONS

Pyloric gland adenoma

These tumours are composed of gastric mucin-producing epithelial cells. They have been found in one series of 3588 gastric polyps (which excluded fundic cystic gland polyps, stromal tumours and lymphomatous polyps) to account for 0.4% of cases.[22] In this series, foci of carcinomatous changes were seen in 40% of these polyps.

Foveolar gland adenoma

These lesions are very rare, can be up to 8 cm in diameter and are mostly found in the body of the stomach (Fig 2.40). The neoplasm is composed entirely of foveolar epithelium with little, or no, stroma (Fig 2.41). They are benign and are not known to be associated with other systemic or localised pathology.[21]

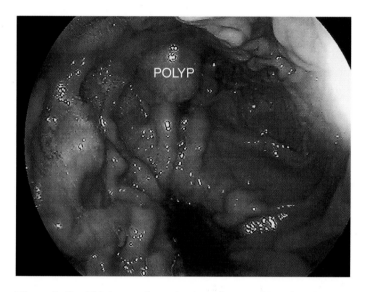

Figure 2.40 – This is an endoscopic view of a case of foveolar adenoma.

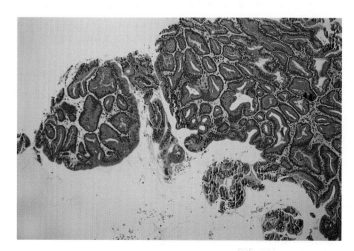

Figure 2.41 – This photomicrograph of foveolar cell adenoma shows proliferation of foveolar cells arranged in an organised fashion in much the same way as occurs in adenomas.

REFERENCES

1. Dekker W: Clinical relevance of gastric and duodenal polyps. *Scand J Gastroenterol* 1990; **25 (supplement 178):** 7–12

2. Niv Y, Bat L: Gastric polyps – a clinical study. *Isr J Med Sci* 1985; **Oct. 21(10):** 841–844

3. Roseau G, Ducreux M, Molas G, *et al*: Epithelial gastric polyps in a series of 13000 gastroscopies. *Presse Med (France)* 1990; **19:** 650–654

4. Owen D: Stomach. In *Histology for Pathologists*, 1st edn, Sternberg SS (ed.). New York, Raven Press 1992: pp. 533–545

5. Saundler F, Hakenson R: Gastric endocrine cell typing at the light microscopy level. In *The Stomach as an Endocrine Organ*, Hakenson R, Saundler F (eds). Amsterdam, Elsevier Science Publishers 1991: pp. 9–26

6. Bordi C, Bertele A, Davighi MC, *et al*: Clinical and pathological association of argyrophilic cell hyperplasia of the gastric mucosa. *Appl Pathol* 1984; **2:** 282–291

7. Fenoglio-Preiser CM, Noffsinger A, Stemmermann GN, *et al* (eds): *Gastrointestinal Pathology; An Atlas and Text*, 2nd edn. Philadelphia, New York, Lippincott-Raven 1998

8. Yamagiwa H, Matsuzaki O, Ishihara A, Yoshimara H: Heterotopic gastritis glands in the submucosa of the stomach. *Acta Pathol Jpn* 1979; **29:** 347–350

9. Heikki J, Jarvinen MD: Other gastrointestinal polyps. *World J Surg* 1991; **15:** 50–56

10. Hizawa K, Iida M, Yak T, Aoyaji K, Fujishima M: Juvenile polyposis of the stomach: clinicopathological features and its malignant potential. *J Clin Pathol* 1997; **50:** 771–774

11. Watanabe H, Jass JR, Sobin LH: *Histological Typing of Oesophageal and Gastric Tumours*. WHO International Classification of Tumours. Berlin, Springer-Verlag 1990

12. Watanabe A, Nagashima H, Motoi M, Ogawa K: Familial juvenile polyposis of the stomach. *Gastroenterology* 1979; **77:** 148–151

13. Ming SC: *Tumours of the Oesophagus and Stomach. Atlas of Tumour Pathology*, 2nd series. Washington, Armed Forces Institute of Pathology 1971

14. Morson BC, Dawson IP, Day DW, Jass JR, Price AB, Williams GT (eds): Benign epithelial polyps. In *Morson & Dawson's Gastrointestinal Pathology*. Oxford, Blackwell Scientific Publication 1991: pp. 351–359

15. Kuwano H, Takana H, Sugimachi K: Solitary Peutz–Jeghers type polyp of the stomach in the absence of familial polyposis coli in a teenage boy. *Endoscopy* 1989; **21:** 188–190

16. Payson BA, Moumgis B: Metastasising carcinoma of the stomach in Peutz–Jeghers syndrome. *Ann Surg* 1967; **165:** 145–151

17. Spigelman AD, Phillips RKS: Peutz–Jeghers syndrome. In *Familial Adenomatous Polyposis and other Polyposis Syndromes*, Phillips RKS, Spigelman AD, Thompson JPS (eds). London, Edward Arnold 1994: pp. 188–202

18. Daniel ES, Ludwig SL, Lewin KJ, Ruprecht RM, Rajalich GM, Schwabe AD: The Cronkhite–Canada syndrome. An analysis of clinical and pathological features and therapy in 55 patients. *Medicine* 1982; **61:** 293–309

19. Day DW, Dixon MF: Gastric polyps and thickened folds. In *Biopsy Pathology of the Oesophagus, Stomach and Duodenum*. London, Chapman and Hall Medical 1995: pp. 171–208

20. Davaris P, Petraki K, Archimandritis A, Haritopoulos N, Papacharalampous N: Mucosal hyperplastic polyps of the stomach. Do they have any potential to malignancy? *J Clin Res* 1986; **4:** 385–389

21. Snover DC: Benign epithelial polyps of the stomach. In *Pathology Annual, vol. 20, Part I*, Somers SC, Rosen PP, Fechner RE (eds). Norwalk, CT, Appleton-Century-Crofts 1985: pp. 303–329

22. Stolte M: Clinical consequences of the endoscopic diagnosis of gastric polyps. *Endoscopy* 1995; **27:** 32–37

23. Mocek FW, Ward WW, Wolfson SE, *et al*: Elimination of recurrent hyperplastic polyps by eradication of *Helicobacter pylori*. *Ann Intern Med* 1994; **120:** 1007–1008

24. Seifer E, Gail K, Weismuller J: Gastric polypectomy – long-term results (survey of 23 centres in Germany). *Endoscopy* 1983; **15:** 8–11

25. Spinelli P, Cerrai FG, Casella G, Calarco G, Clemente C, Pizzetti P: Endoscopic treatment of polyps in the resected stomach. *Minerva Chirurgica* 1994; **49:** 393–396

26. Koch HK, Lesch R, Cremer M, Oelert W: Polyps and polypoid foveolar hyperplasia in gastric biopsy specimens and their precancerous prevalence. *Front Gastrointest Res* 1979; **4:** 183–191

27. Laxen F: Gastric polyps and gastric carcinoma. *Ann Clin Res* 1981; **13:** 154–155

28. Appelman HD: Localised and extensive expansion of the gastric mucosa: mucosal polyps and giant folds. In *Pathology of the Oesophagus, Stomach and Duodenum*, Appelman HD (ed.). New York, Churchill Livingstone 1984: pp. 79–120

29. Orlowska J, Jarosz D, Pachlewski J, Butruk E: Malignant transformation of benign gastric polyps. *Am J Gastroenterol* 1995; **90:** 2152–2159

30. Marcinal MA, Villafana M, Harandez-Denton J, Colon-Pagan JR: The fundic gland polyps: prevalence and clinicopathological features. *Am J Gastroenterol* 1993; **88:** 1711–1713

31. Stolte M, Sticht T, Edit S, Ebert D, Finkenzeller G: Frequency, location, age and sex distribution of various types of gastric polyp. *Endoscopy* 1994; **26:** 656–659

32. Domizio P, Talbot IC, Spigelman AD, Phillips RKS, Williams CB: Upper gastrointestinal tract pathology in familial adenomatous polyposis; results from a prospective study of 102 patients. *J Clin Pathol* 1990; **43:** 738–743

33. Hizawa K, Iida M, Matsumoto T, *et al*: Natural history of fundic gland polyposis without familial adenomatous coli: follow up observation in 31 patients. *Radiology* 1993; **189:** 429–432

34. Iida M, Yao T, Itoh H, *et al*: Natural history of fundic gland polyposis in patients with familial adenomatosis coli/Gardner's syndrome. *Gastroenterology* 1985; **89:** 1021–1025

35. Stolte M, Bethke B, Seifert E, *et al*: Observation of glandular cysts in the corpus mucosa of the stomach under omeprazole treatment. *Z Gastroenterol* 1995; **33:** 146–149

36. Eisenstat D, Griffiths A, Cutz E, *et al*: Acute *cytomegalovirus* infection in a child with Menetrier's disease. *Gastroenterology* 1995; **109:** 592–595

37. Domellof L, Eriksson S, Halender HF, Janunger K-G: Lipid islands in the gastric mucosa after resection for benign ulcer disease. *Gastroenterology* 1977; **72:** 14–18

38. Terruzzi V, Minoli G, Butti GC, Rossini A: Gastric lipid islands in the gastric stump and in non-operated stomach. *Endoscopy* 1980; **12:** 58–62

39. Johnstone JM, Morson BC: Inflammatory fibroid polyp of the gastrointestinal tract. *Histopathology* 1978; **2:** 349–361

40. Stolte M, Finkenzeller G: Inflammatory fibroid polyp of the stomach. *Endoscopy* 1990; **22:** 203–207

41. Kolodziejczyk P, Yao T, Tsuneyoshi M: Inflammatory fibroid polyp of the stomach. A special reference to an immunohistochemical profile of 42 cases. *Am J Surg Pathol* 1993; **17:** 1159–1168

42. Hirota T, Okada T, Itabashi M, *et al*: Histiogenesis of human gastric cancer: with special reference to the significance of adenoma as a precancerous lesion. In *Precursors of Gastric Cancer*, Ming SC (ed.). New York, Praeger Publishers 1984

43. Nagayo T, Ito M, Yakoyama H and Komagoe T: Early phases of human gastric cancer. Morphological study. *(Jpn J Cancer Res) Gann* 1965; **56:** 101–120

44. Tata M, Marakami A, Karita M, Yanai H, Okita K: Endoscopic resection of early gastric cancer. *Endoscopy* 1993; **25:** 445–450

45. Petras RC: Comments of the proceedings of the Endoscopy Master Forum: endoscopy in precancerous, early-stage cancerous conditions of the gastrointestinal tract. *Endoscopy* 1995; **27:** 58–63

46. Ohata H, Noguchi Y, Takagi K, *et al*: Early gastric carcinoma with special reference to macroscopic classification. *Cancer* 1987; **60:** 1099–1106

47. Green PHR, O'Toole KM, Weingberg LM, *et al*: Early gastric cancer. *Gastroenterology* 1981; **81:** 247–256

48. Tsukuma H, Mishima T, Oshima A: Prospective study of early gastric cancer. *Int J Cancer* 1983; **31:** 421–426

49. Kitaoka H, Yoshikawa K, Hirota T, *et al*: Surgical treatment of early gastric cancer. *Jpn J Clin Oncol* 1984; **14:** 283–293

50. Goodwin JD: Carcinoid tumours: an analysis of 2837 cases. *Cancer* 1975; **36:** 560–569

51. Modlin IM, Gilligan CJ, Lawton GP, Tang LH, West B, Darr U: Gastric carcinoids. The Yale Experience. *Arch Surg* 1995; **130:** 250–255

52. Granberg D, Wilander E, Stridsberg M, Graner G, Skogseid B, Oberg K: Clinical symptoms, hormone profiles, treatment and prognosis with gastric carcinoid. *Gut* 1998; **43:** 223–228

53. Davies MG, O'Dowd G, McEntee GP, Hennessy TP: Primary gastric carcinoid, a view on management. *Br J Surg* 1990; **77:** 1013–1014

54. Campbell F, Bogomoletz WV, Williams GT: Tumours of the oesophagus and stomach. In *Diagnostic Histopathology of Tumours*, Fletcher CDM (ed.). Edinburgh, Churchill-Livingstone 1995: pp. 221–224

55. Rosai J: Stromal tumours. In *Ackermans Surgical Pathology*, Rosai J (ed.). St Louis, Boston, Mosby 1995: pp. 645–647

56. McClain KL, Leach CT, Jenson HB, *et al*: Association of Epstein–Barr virus with leiomyosarcomas in young people with AIDS. *N Engl J Med* 1995; **332:** 12–18

57. Raafat F, Salman WD, Roberts K, Ingram L, Rees R, Mann JR: Carney's triad. Gastric leiomyosarcoma, pulmonary chondroma and extra-adrenal paraganglioma in young females. *Histopathology* 1986; **10:** 1325–1333

58. Fiddian RV, Parish JA: Gastric lipomata. *Br J Surg* 1960; **48:** 98–102

59. Chodoff RJ, DeLeon AD: Lipoma of the stomach. *Surgery* 1959; **46:** 841–844

60. Isaacson PG: Gastrointestinal lymphoma. *Hum Pathol* 1994; **25:** 1020–1029

61. Isaacson PG, Maclennan KA, Subbuswamy SG: Multiple lymphomatous polyposis of the gastrointestinal tract. *Histopathology* 1984; **8:** 641–656

62. O'Brien DS, Kennedy MJ, Daly PA, *et al*: 'Multiple lymphomatous polyposis' of the gastrointestinal tract. A clinicopathologically distinctive form of non-Hodgkin's lymphoma, B-cell centrocytic type. *Am J Surg Pathol* 1989; **13:** 691–699

3

Polyps of the Duodenum

NY Haboubi

INTRODUCTION

Upper gastrointestinal (GI) endoscopy should always include examination of the duodenum. The duodenum is different from the rest of the GI tract in the following ways:

- The opening of the biliary and pancreatic ducts in the second part creates a complex macroscopic and histological anatomy with its own pathological entities.

- The complexity of Brunner's glands. These are more dense proximally in the duodenum. Consequently, lesions related to these glands generally occur in the first part of the duodenum.

- Certain polyps have certain anatomical predilections within the duodenum. For example, the commonest duodenal polyps seen at the bulb are of gastric derivatives,[1] while the neoplastic adenomas in patients with familial adenomatous polyposis (FAP) are mostly clustered around the ampullary region.

NORMAL STRUCTURE

Anatomy

The duodenum is the most proximal portion of the small intestine and measures 20–25 cm in length. It extends from the pylorus to the duodeno-jejunal flexure. Most of the organ is fixed. It is situated in the retroperitoneum and forms a 'U' or 'C' shape around the head of the pancreas. Anatomically and endoscopically, it can be divided into the following parts:

- The first part: the duodenal bulb or cap.

- The second part: the descending portion into which the common bile duct and the major and minor pancreatic ducts open.

- The third or horizontal part.

- The fourth or ascending part.

At the end of the fourth part there is the ligament of Treitz, which marks the transition from duodenum to jejunum.

Histology

Like the rest of the small intestine, the duodenal mucosa is characterised by villi. The gastro-duodenal junction, although well defined macroscopically and endoscopically, is in fact poorly demarcated histologically.[2] There is a gradual transition between the two epithelial types, irrespective of the position of the gastro-duodenal junction as characterised by the pyloric musculature. In the proximal duodenum, there are usually three distinct types of epithelium; the small intestinal type, the gastric antral type mucosa and the transitional type.[3] The villi are mostly leaf-like (rather than finger shaped) and are shorter and broader than in the rest of the duodenum, particularly if there is an intramucosal Brunner's gland or overlying lymphoid follicle (Fig 3.1). It is also worth noting that the number of mononuclear cells within the lamina propria is greater in the duodenum in health than in the rest of the small intestine.[4]

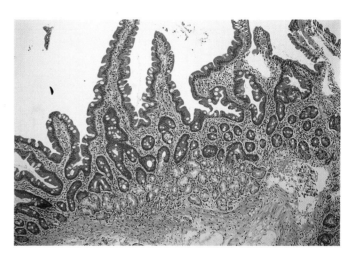

Figure 3.1 – Normal duodenal villi with normal surface epithelium and underlying Brunner's gland, which is very characteristic of the region.

A characteristic histological appearance of the duodenum is the presence of Brunner's glands. Although mostly found in the submucosa, they can also be present in the mucosa. Additionally, they are more concentrated in the first part of the duodenum, becoming scanty in the third and fourth parts. Brunner's glands are lined with cuboidal or columnar cells that have a pale, uniform cytoplasm and oval, basally situated nuclei. The cytoplasm contains periodic acid-Schiff (PAS) +ve diastase resistant neutral mucin. Brunner's glands also contain scattered endocrine cells. The rest of the epithelial cells and the wall are similar to the rest of the small intestine (see Chapter 4 p. 73).

HETEROTOPIC GASTRIC MUCOSA

Synonyms

Duodenal gastric heterotopia.

Prevalence

This may be present in up to 2% of upper GI endoscopies.

Endoscopic appearance

- Usually, the lesion is seen in the first part of the duodenum and is characterised by single or multiple, pink mucosal nodules (Fig 3.2), less than 1 cm in diameter, situated most often on the anterior wall.[5]

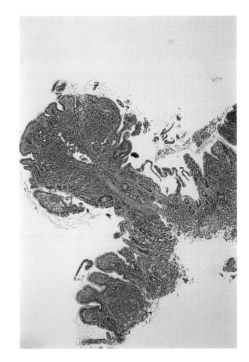

Figure 3.3 – Polypoidal protrusion of gastric tissue in the first part of the duodenum in a case of gastric heterotopia.

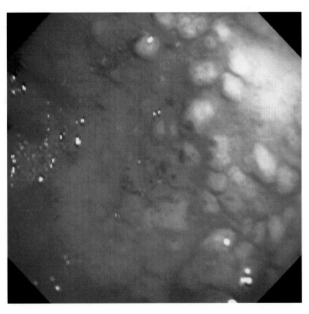

Figure 3.2 – Endoscopic view of heterotopic gastric mucosa. Note the multiple small pink nodules.

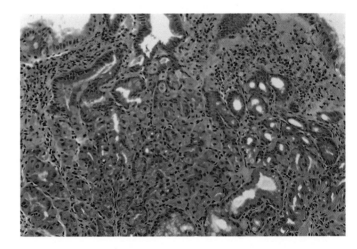

Figure 3.4 – Higher power view of Fig 3.3 showing the body-type gastric acini.

Microscopic features

The characteristic of the lesion is the presence of a collection of orderly gastric glands, ducts and lamina propria (Figs 3.3 & 3.4). The glands have specialised cells, including the chief and parietal cells. The overlying mucosa may be either of gastric or duodenal epithelium.

Gastric heterotopia should not be confused with gastric metaplasia, which is characterised by the presence of gastric (mucin-secreting) cells at the tip of the villi in the first and to a lesser extent the second part of the duodenum. Gastric metaplasia usually appears as a response to acid, especially in association with helicobacter gastritis. It is non-polypoidal and not usually detected endoscopically.

Biological behaviour and associated conditions

The lesions are strictly benign and are not known to have any clinical significance or associated conditions.

Management

No follow-up is required.

HETEROTOPIC PANCREATIC TISSUE

Synonyms

Pancreatic duodenal heterotopia, myoglandular hamartoma, pancreatic adenomyoma.

Prevalence

This is a rare congenital abnormality. It is seen in up to 13.7% of duodenal or jejunal strictures, duplication and Meckel's diverticulum.[6]

The lesion is particularly common in trisomy syndromes especially involving chromosomes 13 and 18.[6]

Endoscopic appearance

- It appears as a sessile, polypoidal elevation sometimes with an umbilicated centre (Fig 3.5).

- It varies in size from a few millimetres to several centimetres in diameter.

- It is almost invariably single and the majority occur 3–4 cm from either side of the pylorus.[7]

Microscopic features

The lesion is composed of pancreatic ducts and acini located in the duodenal submucosa. Islets of Langerhans are seen in approximately one-third of cases.[8]

Sometimes this pancreatic tissue may be accompanied by bundles of hypertrophied smooth muscle surrounding ducts; hence the alternative appellations of adenomyoma and myoglandular hamartoma (Figs 3.6 & 3.7).

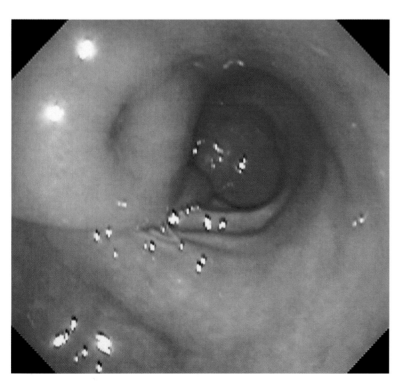

Figure 3.5 – This shows an endoscopic view of heterotopic pancreatic tissue in which there is a slight elevation of the mucosa giving rise to an umbilicated lesion.

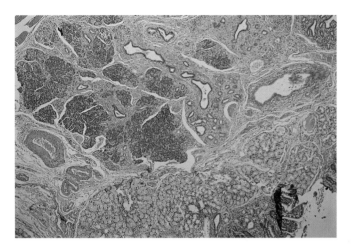

Figure 3.6 – This shows a case of heterotopic pancreatic tissue. Note the pancreatic glands and acini, surrounded by hypertrophied muscle adjacent to Brunner's glands as typically seen in this condition.

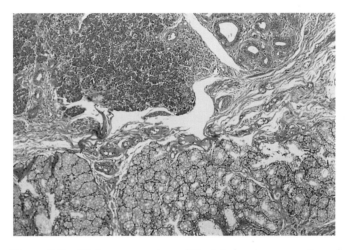

Figure 3.7 – Higher power view of Fig 3.6 showing pancreatic and Brunner's gland tissue.

Biological behaviour and associated conditions

The large lesions nearer the pylorus may produce symptoms of gastric outlet obstruction and, rarely, ulceration and bleeding. Nearer the ampulla, these lesions can produce obstruction of the common bile duct.[9] Nevertheless, it is important to realise that the majority are incidental findings and they produce no clinical symptoms.

Management

In symptomatic patients, endoscopic or simple surgical excision may be required.

BRUNNER'S GLAND HAMARTOMA

Synonyms

Hamartoma.

Prevalence

This is a rare lesion that usually occurs in the fourth to sixth decade of life. The difficulty in ascertaining the true incidence is due to the confusion with Brunner's gland hyperplasia and adenoma.

Endoscopic appearance

- Polypoid smooth nodular lesion usually covered by normal looking mucosa (Fig 3.8).

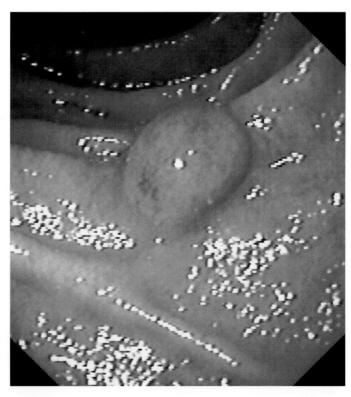

Figure 3.8 – This endoscopic view shows a polypoidal elevated lesion of a case of Brunner's gland hamartoma.

Microscopic features

These lesions have a variable mixture of Brunner's glands and adipose, muscular and pancreatic tissues.

Biological behaviour and associated conditions

They are usually asymptomatic.[10]

On rare occasions they have been reported to cause massive upper GI bleeding.[11]

PEUTZ–JEGHERS POLYPS

Synonyms

See p. 134 in Chapter 6.

Prevalence

The duodenum is sometimes involved in Peutz–Jeghers syndrome. In one study from Japan, which included 222 patients, the duodenum was involved in 47 patients.[12]

Endoscopic appearance

- Polypoidal lesions of variable sizes seen mostly with intact mucosa.

Microscopic features

The histological appearances are similar to those of Peutz–Jeghers polyps in the small intestine and colon (see Chapter 6 p. 135).

In approximately 10% of small intestinal Peutz–Jeghers polyps, there is submucosal herniation or epithelial misplacement (Fig 3.9), which can closely mimic malignant transformation and invasion.[13] This herniation is also called enteritis cystica profunda and is thought to be due to mechanical pressure.[13,14]

Biological behaviour and associated conditions

It has been found that there is a higher risk of malignancy in these polyps than was previously estimated (see p. 136 in Chapter 6).

Management

See p. 136 in Chapter 6.

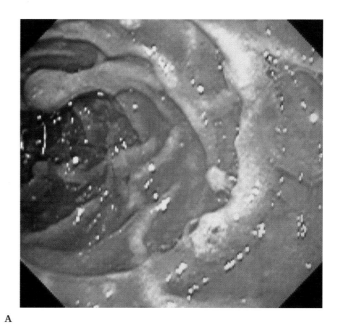

A

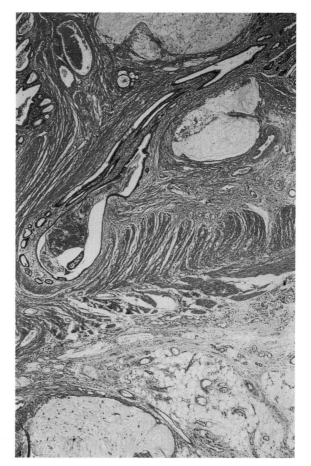

B

Figure 3.9 – (*a*) This shows an endoscopic view of a case of Peutz–Jeghers polyp. (*b*) This shows a case of Peutz–Jeghers syndrome in which there is epithelial herniation into the submucosa. This should not be confused with invasion.

CRONKHITE–CANADA SYNDROME (CCS)

Synonyms

The polyps of juvenile polyposis show superficial similarities to CCS although the polyps of CCS lack the pedunculated nature of colonic juvenile polyps. The two conditions are easily differentiated by the presence of the ectodermal changes of CCS and the very different age distribution.

Prevalence

Duodenal involvement in this syndrome is common. In one study, out of the 29 cases reviewed, there was duodenal involvement in 21 patients.[15]

Endoscopic and gross appearance

- Compared to other polyposis syndromes, the macroscopic changes of CCS appear much more diffuse (Fig 6.11).

- The presence of mucosal cystic change produces a characteristic granular appearance to the mucosa of the stomach and the intestines and there may be gelatinous-appearing polypoid masses.

Management

There is no known active treatment for CCS and management of affected patients is merely supportive. The mortality rate is stated to be about 60%.

JUVENILE POLYPS

Synonyms

Juvenile adenomas (this is a misnomer as there is no evidence of adenomatous change in solitary juvenile polyps in the great majority of cases).

Prevalence

Most of the cases reported so far suggest that the duodenum is affected mostly in cases of juvenile polyposis syndrome and that sporadic juvenile polyps are rare.

Endoscopic appearance

- Although juvenile polyps are usually solitary and most usually demonstrated in the rectum, colonoscopic surveys have shown that they are on occasion multiple (any more than five should raise suspicions of juvenile polyposis (JP)) and evenly distributed throughout the colon.[3]

Microscopic features

The histological appearances of juvenile polyps are not entirely specific and polyps bearing a superficial resemblance to juvenile polyps are seen in inflammatory conditions (inflammatory polyps), at the site of ureterosigmoidostomy,[4] in Cowden's syndrome (see p. 140 in Chapter 6) and in various rarer syndromes.

Biological behaviour and associated conditions

Juvenile polyps usually present with bleeding per rectum. Although sporadic polyps may be multiple, it is important to ensure that there is no evidence of juvenile polyposis, since this is a condition with considerable neoplastic potential (see p. 133 in Chapter 6).

Juvenile polyps themselves have a negligible neoplastic implication. There are only five reports, to our knowledge, documenting dysplastic change within sporadic juvenile polyps[6–11] and two cases describing carcinoma arising in solitary juvenile polyps.[12,13]

BRUNNER'S GLAND HYPERPLASIA

Synonyms

Brunner's gland adenoma.

Prevalence

These are rare lesions.

Endoscopic appearance

Two forms have been described:

- The first type is composed of single or multiple, discrete, circumscribed, sessile polyps that mostly affect the first part of the duodenum (Fig 3.10).

- The second type is a more diffuse process affecting mainly the more distal part of the duodenum and in which there is cobblestone nodular elevations of the mucosa.[16]

Microscopic features

Characterized by the presence of clusters of normal Brunner's gland separated by thin fibrovascular stroma (including strands of smooth muscle from the muscularis mucosae) (Fig 3.11). On occasion, there may be some lymphocytic aggregates.

It is important to remember that a small or superficial endoscopic biopsy may not be helpful in making such a diagnosis.

Biological behaviour and associated conditions

Can be seen in isolation or in association with *either* acid hypersecretion, chronic renal failure *or* chronic duodenitis.[17]

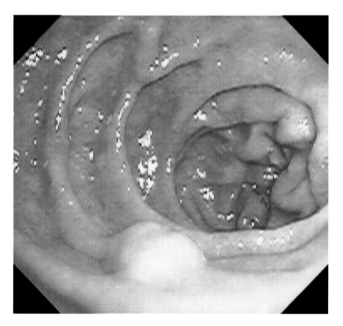

Figure 3.10 – This shows an endoscopic view of Brunner's gland hyperplasia/adenoma.

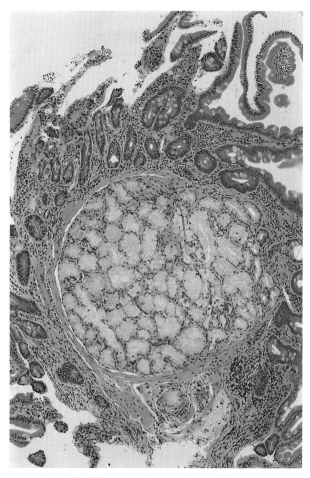

Figure 3.11 – This illustrates a Brunner's gland hyperplasia/adenoma showing the proliferation of Brunner's gland surrounded by a rim of muscular tissue.

These lesions are usually benign. Only very occasional examples of malignant lesions arising from Brunner's glands have been described.[18]

Management

Endoscopic polypectomy is a sufficient treatment and no follow-up is required.

NODULAR LYMPHOID HYPERPLASIA

Synonyms

Follicular lymphoid hyperplasia, diffuse follicular lymphoid hyperplasia.

Prevalence

The duodenum is rarely affected by this disorder.

Endoscopic appearance

- They appear as multiple, small, sessile mucosal elevations.

Microscopic features

The lesions manifest themselves as nodules of dense lymphocytic infiltrate with formation of follicles (usually with germinal centres) (Fig 3.12).

These nodules are characteristically located in the lamina propria and are covered by a single layer of enterocytes.

Sometimes the nodules extend into the submucosa.

The villi and crypts are short or absent in the lymphoid areas but are normal in between.

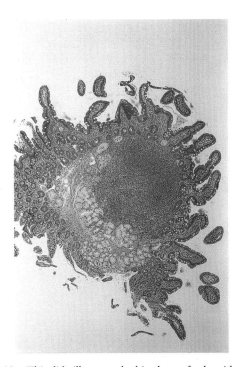

Figure 3.12 – This slide illustrates the histology of polypoidal hyperplasia of the lymphoid tissue, where there is proliferation of the lymphocytes abutting on Brunner's gland. Sometimes there are prominent germinal centres.

Biological behaviour and associated conditions

Although there is an association with acquired idiopathic hypogammaglobulinaemia (AIH), the majority of patients with that disorder do not have NLH.[19]

Patients with AIH who have NLH *may* have Giardiasis, chronic diarrhoea or intestinal lymphoma.[20,21]

Management

Variable; in most patients there is a need for medical treatment for the *Giardia*.

Sometimes, there is a need for supportive therapy. A low fat diet has been suggested.[21]

ADENOMAS

Synonyms

Adenomatous polyp, villous adenoma, tubular adenoma, tubulovillous adenoma.

Prevalence

Adenomas of the duodenum are rare sporadic lesions. However nearly all patients with familial adenomatous polyposis (FAP) have duodenal adenomas[22] (see p. 125 in Chapter 6).

Endoscopic appearance

- Adenomatous polyps vary in size from microscopic to large neoplasms occupying most of the lumen (Fig 3.13).

- Some adenomas are sessile whilst others are pedunculated.

- In patients with FAP, the distribution is characteristically around and beyond the papilla[23] and is thought to be related to the degree of mucosal exposure to bile. In one series[23] of 88 patients, none had adenomas of the bulb alone, 10% had involvement of the bulb and of the 2nd and 3rd parts, whilst 90% of the patients had involvement of the 2nd and 3rd parts only.

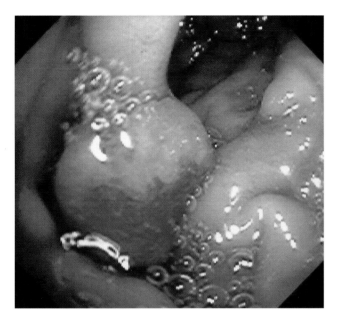

Figure 3.13 – Endoscopic view of tubular adenoma.

Microscopic features

As with its colonic counterpart, the architecture of duodenal adenoma can be tubular, tubulovillous or villous with varying degrees of dysplasia (Fig 3.14).

Micro-adenomas have also been noted in the endoscopically normal appearing mucosa in patients with FAP.

Unlike the colon however, the presence of neoplastic epithelial elements invading the lamina propria is a strong indication of malignancy, since the great majority of adenomas showing intramucosal carcinomas at biopsy will exhibit deeper invasion in the resected specimens.[17]

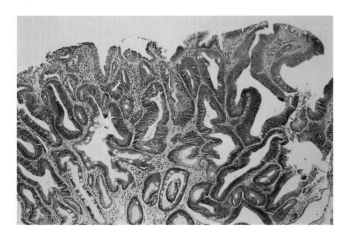

Figure 3.14 – Microscopic view of tubulovillous adenoma of the duodenum. Note the similarity to its colonic counterpart.

In the ampullary region the distinction between adenoma and well differentiated adenocarcinoma can be very difficult. This is due to the fact that small glands can be surrounded by muscle bundles under normal conditions. This feature should not be mistaken for invasion.

Biological behaviour and associated conditions

In patients with FAP, there is strong evidence to support the adenoma-carcinoma sequence.[22] In a large series, adenomatous tissue was found within duodenal cancer in 66% of cases and in mucosa adjacent to duodenal cancer in 73% of cases.

It appears that villous architecture, high grade dysplasia and the high volume of polyps are markers for malignant change within an individual polyp and elsewhere in the duodenum.[22]

Management

The treatment for a sporadic single polyp is polypectomy. Some advocate transduodenal excisions.[25]

In patients with FAP, polypectomy has resulted in recurrence in all 12 patients reported in one series.[24] The authors concluded that 'local excision of duodenal adenomas is an unsatisfactory treatment option in those with FAP and that the ideal management with severe duodenal polyposis remains uncertain'.

Treatment with the non-steroidal anti-inflammatory drug sulindac has shown a 'trend' in duodenal polyp regression and a reduction in epithelial cell proliferation[26] (see p. 130 in Chapter 6). However, one other study found it to be of no benefit.[27]

Some centres have suggested Whipple's operation for patients with duodenal FAP but others cautioned against even surveillance, arguing that, in their large series, it only increases life expectancy by 7 months.[28]

ADENOCARCINOMA

Synonyms

Papillary adenocarcinoma.

Prevalence

In general, duodenal carcinoma is an uncommon tumour comprising about 0.3% of all gastrointestinal neoplasms.[17]

Endoscopic appearance

- Most cases appear in the periampullary region and therefore it is often difficult to distinguish between biliary, pancreatic, ampullary and duodenal carcinoma, especially in the late stages of the disease (Figs 3.15 & 3.16).

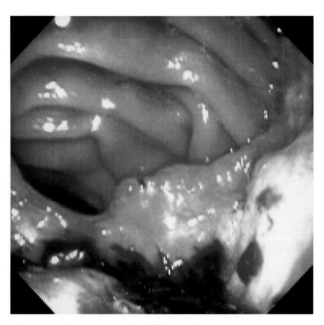

Figure 3.15 – An endoscopic view of duodenal adenocarcinoma.

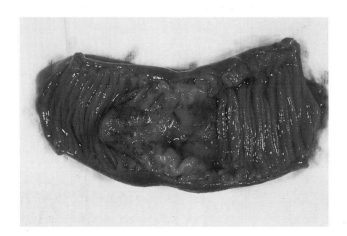

Figure 3.16 – Gross appearance of a surgical specimen with adenocarcinoma of the duodenum.

Microscopic features

Like adenocarcinoma in the stomach and colon (Fig 3.17), there is a variable degree of differentiation. The cell population may include absorptive, secretory and, to a lesser extent, Paneth and endocrine cells.

It is common to see an adenomatous component, emphasising the adenoma–carcinoma sequence.[29]

Biological behaviour and associated conditions

The most important association is with FAP. It is estimated that the vast majority of FAP patients will develop duodenal adenomas.[22] A significant proportion will progress to carcinoma. Indeed duodenal carcinoma has now become the commonest cause of death in the syndrome.

Coeliac disease is also a predisposing factor for duodenal adenocarcinoma, which is normally preceded by adenoma formation.[30,31]

The outcome depends on the stage of the disease and the location and size of the tumour.

Management

Surgery is the treatment of choice for curative therapy.

In palliative therapy, endoscopic laser treatment has been suggested as an option.[32]

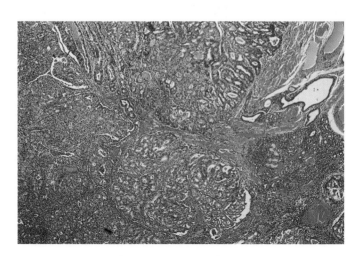

Figure 3.17 – Microphotograph of adenocarcinoma. Note the similarity to colonic adenocarcinoma.

NEUROENDOCRINE TUMOURS

Synonyms

Carcinoids, endocrine tumours.

Prevalence

In general, duodenal carcinoids account for 1–2.3% of all gastrointestinal carcinoids.[36]

Most tumours occur in the first and second parts of the duodenum.[33,34]

The neoplasm occurs slightly more frequently in males with an average age of about 60.[34]

Only one in five duodenal carcinoids will be polypoid.[35]

Endoscopic appearance

- The neoplasms may be single or multiple.

- They are often misinterpreted as gastric or pancreatic heterotopia.

- They have a characteristic smooth elevation, with an irregular shaped erythematous depression or ulceration (Fig 3.18).[36]

- The size varies between 0.2–5 cm but most are less than 2 cm in diameter.[34]

- In some gastrinomas, the neoplasms are microscopic and are therefore not apparent endoscopically.[37]

Microscopic features

These neoplasms have a monomorphic appearance of solid and sometimes anastomosing ribbons (Fig 3.19). Characteristically, they stain with Grimelius and with immunohistochemical stains for peptides such as gastrin, vasoactive intestinal peptide (VIP), glucagon and catecholamine.[33]

A special subtype, associated with von Recklinghausen's disease and pheochromocytomas, is characterised by the presence of psammoma bodies and micro-glandular differ-

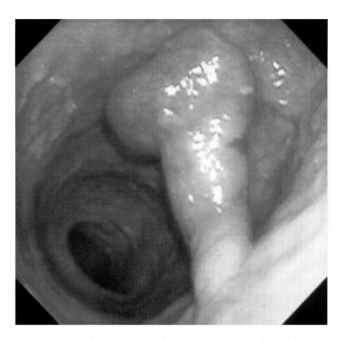

Figure 3.18 – Endoscopic view of a neuroendocrine polypoidal tumour.

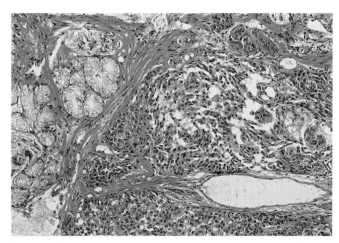

Figure 3.19 – Microphotograph of a neuroendocrine tumour. Note the typically monotonous cells arranged in uniform acinar structures.

entiation.[38] These tumours stain positively with somatostatin.

Biological behaviour and associated conditions

Most duodenal carcinoids do not produce endocrine symptoms.[17]

Approximately 80% of duodenal carcinoids are benign.[34]

Some, however, are associated with the Zollinger–Ellison syndrome, gastrinoma and multiple endocrine neoplasia (MEN)-type I syndrome[37] (pituitary adenoma, parathyroid hyperplasia and island cell tumour of the pancreas). Others are associated with phaeochromocytoma.[39] The latter is almost always situated in the ampullary region, often having invasive tendencies.[39]

In a series of 99 cases of duodenal carcinoid,[34] malignancy was related to the following factors:

- Size: no metastasis was seen in tumours less than 2 cm in diameter.

- Mitotic counts.

- Invasion of the muscularis propria.

Management

Surgery is the treatment of choice.

However, if the patient's condition and tumour location precludes surgical removal, endoscopic stripping of neoplasms that are less than 1 cm in diameter and confined to the mucosa is an acceptable alternative.[36]

GANGLIOCYTIC PARAGANGLIOMAS

Synonyms

Benign non-chromaffin paragangliomas, stromal tumours of neural origin, neuroendocrine tumours.

Prevalence

A very rare tumour: only a few cases have been reported in the literature.[40–43]

They are mostly seen in men.[40]

Endoscopic/gross appearance

- They appear as circumscribed polypoidal lesions up to 5 cm in diameter.[41]

- They are seen mostly in the medial aspect of the second part of the duodenum around the ampulla of Vater.

Microscopic features

Contain a mixture of clusters of columnar epithelium intermixed with spindle cell components that can have the typical features of neurofibroma or Schwannoma (Figs 3.20 & 3.21) and cells with the appearances of ganglion cells.

A reticulin stain is useful for demonstrating the triphasic nature of these lesions.

Biological behaviour and associated conditions

These are benign tumours. One case has been reported to be associated with somatostatin-rich carcinoid in a patient with von Recklinghausen's disease.[42] The usual presenting

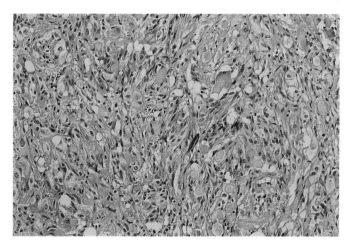

Figure 3.20 – Low power microphotograph view of gangliocytic paraganglioma.

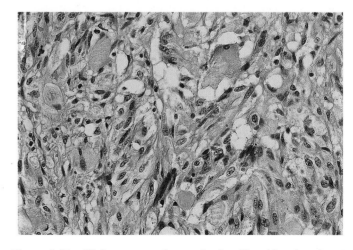

Figure 3.21 – Higher power microscopic view illustrating the mixture of cells including ganglia.

features are nausea, gastrointestinal bleeding, vomiting and obstructive jaundice when the lesion involves the ampulla of Vater.[43]

The neoplasms are thought to be a hybrid between ganglio-cytoma and non-chromaffin paraganglioma.

Management

All cases reported so far are benign and therefore local surgery is suggested for symptomatic patients.

STROMAL POLYPS

Synonyms

Smooth muscle tumours, spindle cell tumours.

Prevalence

In general stromal tumours in the duodenum occur with a frequency that is out of all proportion to the length of the duodenum compared with the rest of the small intestine.

Roughly 60% arise in the second part, 25% in the first part and 15% in both the third and fourth parts.[44]

Endoscopic appearance

- They appear as raised, usually solitary, nodules with smooth covering mucosa (Fig 3.22).

- Sometimes they have a central area of ulceration.

- The malignant lesions are usually greater than 5 cm in diameter.[45]

Microscopic features

Benign lesions are composed of uniform spindle cells with low cellularity and mitotic figures of 2 or less/50 high power fields (HPF) (Fig 3.23).

Malignant lesions are more cellular, pleomorphic and show 2 or more mitotic figures/50 HPF.

They stain positive for vimentin, some for S100 protein and others for CD34. Once again the unifying hypothesis of GISTs, related to CD117 expression, is emphasised (see pp. 45–46).

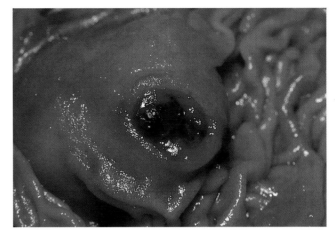

Figure 3.22 – Endoscopic view of benign stromal tumour.

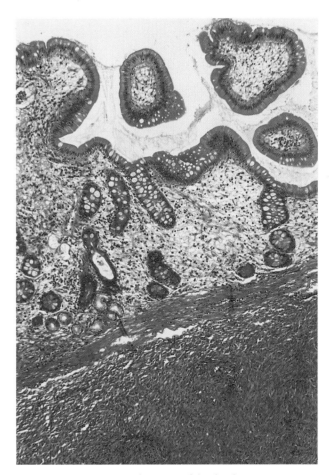

Figure 3.23 – Benign stromal tumour of the duodenum.

Biological behaviour and associated conditions

Malignant lesions have a poor prognosis.[45]

Management

Radical surgery for malignant tumours.

REFERENCES

1. Matsui K, Kitagawa M: Biopsy study of polyps in the duodenal bulb. *Am J Gastroenterol* 1993; **88:** 253–257

2. Lawson HH: The duodenal mucosa in health and disease. A clinical and experimental study. *Surg Annu* 1989; **21:** 157–180

3. Lawson HH: Definition of the gastro-duodenal junction in healthy subjects. *J Clin Pathol* 1988; **41:** 393–396

4. Goldman H, Antonoli DA: Mucosal biopsy of the oesophagus, stomach and proximal duodenum. *Hum Pathol* 1982; **13(5):** 423–448

5. Lessells AM, Martin D: Heterotopic gastric mucosa in the duodenum. *J Clin Pathol* 1982; **35:** 591–595

6. The neoplastic stomach. In *Gastrointestinal pathology; an atlas and text*, 2nd edn, Fenoglio-Preiser CM, Noffsinger A, Stemmermann GN, *et al* (eds). Philadelphia, Lippincott-Raven 1998: pp. 237–274

7. Zarlig EJ: Gastric adenomyoma with coincidental pancreatic arrest. A case report. *Gastrointest Endosc* 1981; **27:** 175–177

8. Nickels J, Laasonen EM: Pancreatic heterotopia. *Scand J Gastroenterol* 1970; **5:** 639–640

9. Bill K, Belber JP, Carson JW: Adenomyoma of the duodenum producing common bile duct obstruction. *Gastrointest Endosc* 1982; **28:** 182–184

10. Tsujimura T, Arai K, Tanaka M, *et al*: Endoscopic removal of recurrent duodenal hamartoma. *Endoscopy* 1993; **25:** 545–546

11. Kouraklis G, Kostakis A, Delladestima J: Hamartoma of Brunner's glands causing massive haematemesis. *Scand J Gastroenterol* 1994; **29:** 841–843

12. Utsunomiya J, Gosh H, Miyagi T, *et al*: Peutz–Jeghers syndrome: its natural course and management. *Johns Hopkins Med J* 1975; **136:** 71–82

13. Shepherd NA, Bussey HJR, Jass JR: Epithelial misplacement in Peutz–Jeghers polyps: a diagnostic pitfall. *Am J Surg Pathol* 1987; **11:** 743–749

14. Kyriakos M, Condon SC: Enteritis cystica profunda. *Am J Clin Pathol* 1978; **69:** 77–85

15. Qizilibash AH: Epithelial neoplasms of the duodenum and periampullary region. In *Pathology of the oesophagus, stomach and duodenum*, Appelman HD (ed.). New York, Churchill-Livingstone 1984: pp. 145–174

16. Merine D, Jones B, Ghahramani GG, Hamilton SR, Bayless TM: Hyperplasia of Brunner's gland; the spectrum of its radiographic manifestation. *Gastrointest Radiol* 1991; **16:** 104–108

17. Day DW, Dixon MF: Non-neoplastic polyps and tumours of the duodenum. In *Biopsy pathology of the oesophagus, stomach and duodenum*, 2nd edn, Day DW, Dixon MF (eds). London, Chapman & Hall Medical 1995; pp. 279–302

18. Itsuno M, Makiyama K, Omagari K, *et al*: Carcinoma of the duodenal bulb arising from the Brunner's gland. *Gastroenterol Jpn* 1993; **28:** 118–125

19. Ajdukiewicz AB, Youngs GR, Bouchier IAD: Nodular lymphoid hyperplasia with hypogammaglobulinaemia. *Gut* 1972; **13:** 589–595

20. Hermans PE, Diaz-Buxo KA, Stobo JD: Idiopathic late-onset immunoglobulin deficiency. *Am J Med* 1976; **61:** 221–237

21. Rambaud JC, de Saint-Louvent P, Marti R, *et al*: Diffuse follicular lymphoid hyperplasia of the small intestine without primary immunoglobulin deficiency. *Am J Med* 1982; **73:** 125–132

22. Spigelman AD, Talbot IC, Penna C, *et al*: The evidence for adenoma-carcinoma sequence in duodenum of patients with familial adenomatous polyposis. *J Clin Pathol* 1994; **47:** 709–710

23. Spigelman AD, Williams CB, Talbot IC, Domizio P, Phillips RKS: Upper gastrointestinal cancer in patients with familial adenomatous polyposis. *Lancet* 1989; **ii:** 783–785

24. Sand JA, Nordback IH: Transduodenal excision of benign adenoma of the papilla of Vater. *Euro J Surg* 1995; **161:** 269–275

25. Penna C, Phillips RKS, Tiret E, Spigelman AD: Surgical polypectomy of duodenal adenomas in familial adenomatous polyposis: experience of two European centres. *Br J Surg* 1993; **80:** 1027–1029

26. Nugent KP, Farmer KCR, Spigelman AD, Williams CB, Phillips RKS: Randomised controlled trial to the effect of sulindac on duodenal and rectal polyposis and cell proliferation in patients with familial adenomatous polyposis. *Br J Surg* 1993; **80:** 1618–1619

27. Richard CS, Berk T, Bapat BV, *et al*: Sulindac for periampullary polyps in FAP patients. *Int J Colorect Dis* 1997; **12:** 14–18

28. Vasen HFA, Bulow S, Myrhoj T, *et al*: Decision analysis in the management of duodenal adenomatosis in familial adenomatous polyposis. *Gut* 1997; **40:** 716–719

29. Perzin KH, Bridge MF: Adenomas of the small intestine; a clinicopathological preview of 51 cases and a study of their relationship to carcinoma. *Cancer* 1981; **48:** 799–819

30. Holmes GKT, Dunn GI, Cockel R, Brooks VS: Adenocarcinoma of the upper small bowel complicating coeliac disease. *Gut* 1980; **21:** 1010–1016

31. Fishman MJ, Jeejeebhoy KN, Gopinath N, *et al*: Small intestinal villous adenoma and coeliac disease. *Am J Gastroenterol* 1990; **85:** 748–751

32. Laukku MA, Wang KK: Endoscopic ND: YAG laser palliation of malignant duodenal tumours. *Gastrointest Endosc* 1995; **41:** 225–229

33. Martin ED, Potet F: Pathology of endocrine tumours of the GI tract. *Clin Gastroenterol* 1974; **3(3):** 511–532

34. Burke A, Sobin LH, Federspiel BH, Shekitka KM, Helwig EB: Carcinoid tumours of the duodenum. *Arch Path Lab Med* 1990; **114:** 700–704

35. Willander E, Grimelius L, Lundquist G, Skooj V: Polypeptide hormones in Argentaffin, Argyrophil gastroduodenal endocrine tumours. *Am J Pathol* 1979; **96:** 519–530

36. Peng CL, Lin HJ, Wang K, Lai CR, Lee SD: Treatment of duodenal carcinoid by strip biopsy. *J Clin Gasteroenterol* 1995; **20(2):** 168–172

37. Pipeleers-Marichal M, Somers G, Willems G, *et al*: Gastrinomas in the duodenum of patients with multiple endocrine neoplasia type I and the Zollinger–Ellison syndrome. *New Engl J Med* 1990; **322:** 723–727

38. Griffiths DFR, Williams GT, Williams ED: Multiple endocrine neoplasia associated with von Recklinghausen's disease. *Br Med J* 1983; **287:** 1341–1343

39. Dayal Y, Nunnemacher G, Doos WA, *et al*: Psammomatous somatostatinomas of the duodenum. *Am J Surg Pathol* 1983; **7:** 653–665

40. Taylor HB, Helwig EB: Benign non-chromaffin paraganglioma of the duodenum. *Virch Arch Path Anat* 1962; **335:** 356–366

41. Keps JJ, Zacharias DL: Gangliocytic paragangliomas of the duodenum. A report of two cases with light and electron microscopy examination. *Cancer* 1971; **27:** 61–70

42. Stephens M, Williams GT, Jasani B, Williams ED: Synchronous duodenal neuroendocrine tumour in von Recklinghausen's disease: a case report of gangliocytic paraganglioma and stomatostatin rich glandular carcinoid. *Histopathology* 1987; **11:** 1331–1340

43. Scheithauer BW, Nora FE, Lechago J, *et al*: Duodenal gangliocytic paraganglioma. Clinicopathologic and immunohistochemical study of 11 cases. *Am J Clin Pathol* 1986; **86:** 559–567

44. Appelman HD: Stromal tumours of the oesophagus. In *Pathology of the oesophagus, stomach and duodenum*. New York, Churchill-Livingstone 1984: pp. 195–242

45. Goldblum JR, Appelman HD: Stromal tumours of the duodenum: a histologic and immunohistochemical study of 20 cases. *Am J Surg Pathol* 1995; **1:** 71–80

Polyps of the Jejunum and Ileum

K Geboes and N Ectors

INTRODUCTION

Small intestinal polyps and neoplasms are rare, constituting less than 2% of all gastrointestinal tumours. The diagnosis is usually made by radiological examination. Endoscopic exploration is potentially of prime importance for macroscopic diagnosis and histology. For submucosal lesions, such as stromal tumours, endoscopic biopsies may fail to provide a diagnosis because of their limited size. Endoscopic treatment is possible for some lesions (especially those that are pedunculated). Nevertheless, surgery is needed in most cases that require removal. Surgery and/or chemotherapy is indicated for lymphomas and as an adjuvant therapy for some other lesions.

NORMAL STRUCTURE

Normal structure

Anatomy

Grossly the small intestine is divided somewhat arbitrarily into the duodenum, jejunum and ileum. The jejunum begins at the duodeno-jejunal flexure. Its origin is marked externally by a thickening of the mesentery (a strip of fibromuscular tissue) called the ligament of Treitz. This anchors the terminal duodenum to the posterior abdominal wall. The jejunum constitutes 40% of the small intestine and the ileum makes up the remainder, ending distally at the ileocaecal valve. The structure and function of the jejunum and ileum are substantially different. The differences occur gradually so a clear anatomical or functional localisation of a precise jejuno-ileal transition zone is impossible.

Several architectural adaptations augment the surface of the small intestine. One of these is the folds of Kerckring (plicae circulares) that increase the surface area. These mucosa-covered folds contain submucosal cores. Their orientation is perpendicular to the longitudinal axis of the bowel. They are most prominent between the mid-duodenum and jejunum, widely separated in the proximal ileum and absent in the distal ileum.

Histology

As in the other segments of the gastrointestinal tract, the wall of the small bowel can be divided into four basic layers:

mucosa, submucosa, muscularis externa (or propria) and serosa. The mucosa is composed of epithelium, connective tissue (or lamina propria) and muscularis mucosae (Fig 4.1). The epithelium and lamina propria form the basic structure of intraluminal projections (called villi) and crypts. The villi appear to be tall and of even width. The epithelium (a layer that is a single cell thick and is composed of columnar cells lining the crypts and covering the villi) can be divided into several compartments. The villous epithelium consists of mature, differentiated cells. The absorptive cell is the main type. It is a tall, columnar cell with a basally located nucleus and a brush border at the apical surface. Interspersed among the absorptive cells are goblet cells and scanty endocrine cells. The crypt zone consists of a mixture of immature (stem) cells, goblet, absorptive, Paneth and a large variety of endocrine cells. Paneth cells (normally found only in the crypts) comprise most of the base of individual crypts. The

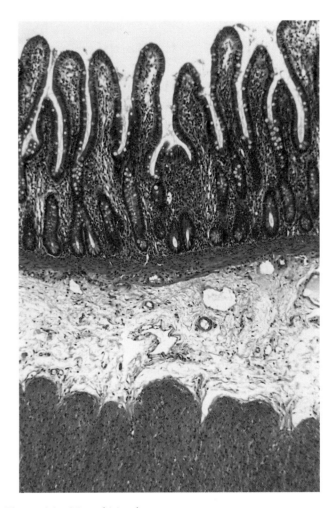

Figure 4.1 – Normal jejunal type mucosa.

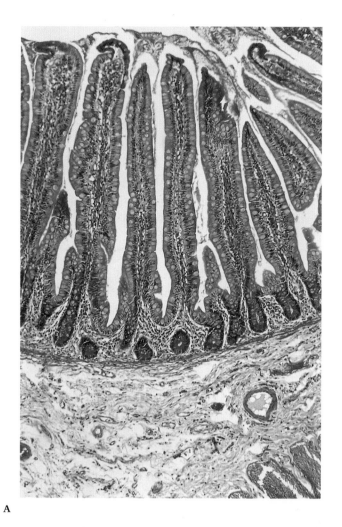

A

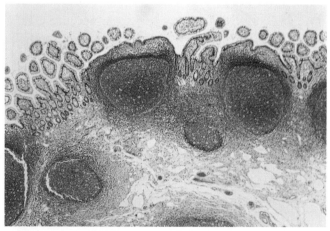

B

Figure 4.2 – (*a*) Normal ileal type mucosa. (*b*) Normal ileal mucosa with Peyer's patches.

surface epithelium is in a state of rapid renewal with each cell having a life span of approximately 5 days. Lymphocytes are present in the surface and crypt epithelium.

The most conspicuous feature of the lamina propria is its abundant immunocompetent and migratory cell component. Five types of immunocompetent cells are normally encountered: mast cells, eosinophils, histiocytes, lymphocytes and plasma cells. Lymphoid follicles in the lamina propria appear as dome-shaped protrusions. They may be single or occur in groups as Peyer's patches (Fig 4.2). The latter are large and numerous in the ileum and are located on the anti-mesenteric border. They are smaller and fewer in the jejunum.

The submucosa is a loose paucicellular layer of fibrous tissue between the muscularis mucosae and the muscularis propria. Relatively large calibre arterioles, venules, lymphatics and neural structures form extensive networks (or plexuses) within this layer. The muscularis externa is composed of an outer, longitudinally running layer and an inner circular band. In between lies a fibrous septum with the myenteric plexus of Auerbach. The muscularis is covered externally by subserosal connective tissue and serosa.[1,2]

HETEROTOPIAS

Prevalence

Heterotopic gastric mucosa in the small intestine, other than in either the duodenum or in congenital anomalies (e.g. Meckel's diverticulum), is exceedingly rare. The jejunum is the most common site.[3]

Heterotopic pancreatic tissue can occur in the jejunum (28% in a series of 272 heterotopic lesions) and in the ileum (10%).[4]

Macroscopic appearance

- The aberrant gastric mucosa forms polypoid, nodular or rugose masses.[5]

- Pancreatic heterotopias are submucosal tumour-like masses usually 3–20 mm in diameter.

Microscopic features

Histologically, mucous and gastric glands with chief and parietal cells and overlying foveolar mucosa are seen (Fig

4.3). An occasional case of a gastric hyperplasiogenic polyp has been described in an inverted Meckel's diverticulum.[6]

In pancreatic heterotopia exocrine pancreatic glands, excretory ducts and islets of Langerhans may both be present. A relative excess of dilated ductal elements and atrophy of glands may make identification difficult.

Biological behaviour and associated conditions

Heterotopic gastric mucosa may ulcerate, bleed, or cause intussusception.[5]

Pancreatic heterotopias are most often discovered as an incidental finding.

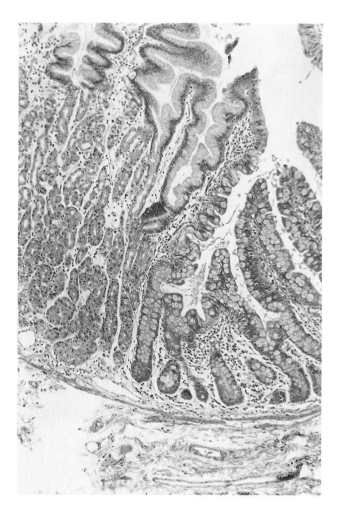

Figure 4.3 – High power view of a small intestinal biopsy with gastric heterotopia appearing as an elevated pseudotumoral lesion. The gastric mucosa is a normal fundic type mucosa with foveolar hyperplasia in the transition zone, towards the small intestine.

Management

No follow-up is needed after initial polypectomy.

HAMARTOMATOUS POLYP

Synonyms

Myoepithelial hamartoma, polypoid hamartoma.

Prevalence

Multiple lesions can be part of either a familial (Peutz–Jeghers syndrome, juvenile polyposis syndrome, Cowden's disease etc Chapter 6) or a non-familial intestinal polyposis (Cronkhite–Canada syndrome: see Chapter 6).

Occasionally a solitary lesion is seen within the small intestine in otherwise normal patients.[7–9]

Macroscopic appearance

- The polyps in Peutz–Jeghers may be sessile or pedunculated, show a lobulated surface and may resemble adenomas (Fig 4.4).

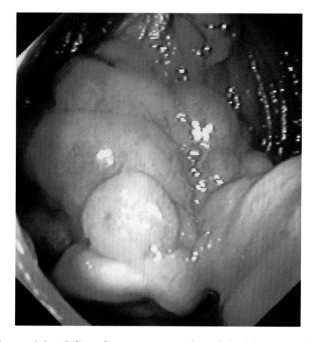

Figure 4.4 – Solitary hamartomatous polyp of the jejunum: sessile, round lesion with smooth surface.

Microscopic features

Histologically, Peutz-Jeghers polyps show a branching stalk of smooth muscle covered by a single layer of normal epithelium (Fig 4.5).

Biological behaviour and associated conditions

Peutz–Jeghers polyps are regarded as having a 'malignant potential'.[10] An increased incidence of gastrointestinal cancer, especially colorectal, has been reported in patients with juvenile polyposis syndrome.

Management

Resection, either surgically or endoscopically, is indicated in symptomatic cases.[11]

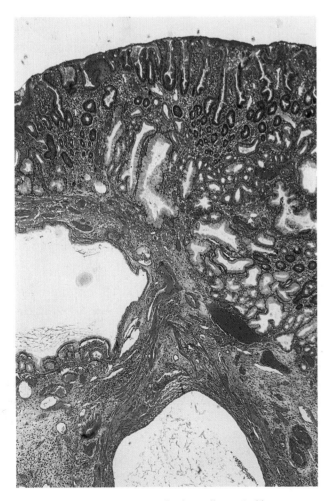

Figure 4.5 – Low power photograph of a small intestinal hamartomatous polyp with hyperplastic crypts and irregular smooth muscle tissue.

INFLAMMATORY FIBROID POLYPS

Synonyms

Fibrous inflammatory polyps, eosinophilic granulomas.

Prevalence

Inflammatory fibroid polyps (IFPs) of the small bowel are rare lesions, usually located in the (terminal) ileum.

They differ from gastric IFPs by being larger, more frequently pedunculated and ulcerated.

Patients are typically older women.[12]

IFPs can occur in association with Crohn's disease.[13]

Macroscopic appearance

- Most of the lesions appear as large (median = 4 cm), intramural, egg-shaped or plaque-like masses or polyps, firm or rubbery in consistency and white, yellow or pink in colour (Fig 4.6).

- Ulceration is common.[14]

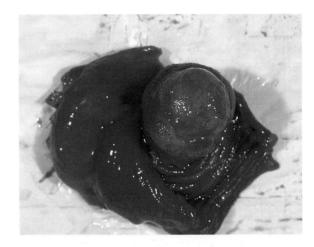

Figure 4.6 – Surgical specimen of the ileum containing a large pedunculated inflammatory fibroid polyp, superficially eroded.

Microscopic features

The lesion originates in the submucosa but often infiltrates the muscularis propria (Fig 4.7). The bulk of the lesion is made up of spindle-shaped or stellate cells without nuclear atypia associated with inflammatory cells (Fig 4.8).

Eosinophils may be predominant but lymphocytes, plasma cells and mast cells are usually present. Blood vessels are numerous.

Occasionally proliferative foci with many mitoses and nuclear hyperchromatism can be seen. Superficially,[14,15] these foci can resemble sarcoma.

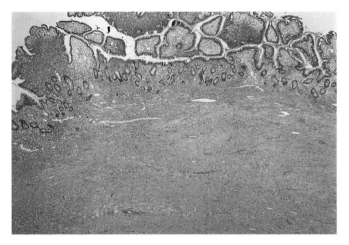

Figure 4.7 – Microscopic examination of the specimen shown in Fig 4.6 demonstrated the presence of a fibrovascular stroma with a diffuse inflammatory reaction, partially covered by atrophic intestinal mucosa. The lesion arises in the submucosa.

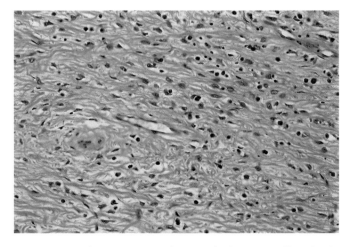

Figure 4.8 – Higher power magnification of inflammatory fibroid polyp showing dense fibrosis, vascular proliferation and chronic inflammatory cell infiltrate.

Biological behaviour and associated conditions

These are invariably benign lesions.

Symptoms are usually non-specific and include abdominal colicky pain as well as intestinal obstruction due to intussusception.

Anaemia and gross bleeding have occasionally been reported.[12,16]

Management

Surgical treatment is indicated for symptomatic lesions.

GRANULATION TISSUE POLYPS

Synonyms

Inflammatory polyps.

Prevalence

Rare.

Macroscopic appearance

- Pale brown, sessile or larger pedunculated lesions.[17,18]

Microscopic features

The lesion consists of a proliferation, to variable degrees, of capillaries, smooth muscle cells, fibroblasts and inflammatory cells (Fig 4.9).

Biological behaviour and associated conditions

These lesions are essentially benign and can occur in the ileum in association with inflammatory conditions (such as Crohn's disease) and, less frequently, with intestinal infections (such as *Yersinia enterocolitica*).[18,19] They are also described as a complication of stricturing malignant carcinoid tumours of the small bowel.[17]

Management

No special treatment is needed.

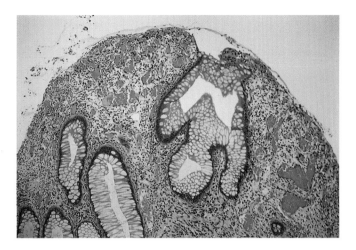

Figure 4.9 – Microscopic appearance of a granulation tissue polyp showing ulcerating surface epithelium, dilated crypts and the congested stroma, which is dense and contains the mixed inflammatory cell infiltrates that are typical of granulation tissue.

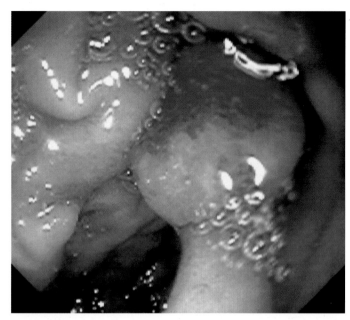

Figure 4.10 – Pedunculated adenomas of the small intestine are rare. The endoscopic appearance is similar to that of pedunculated adenomas in the colon.

ADENOMAS

Synonyms

Polypoid benign glandular tumours.

Prevalence

Although rare, genuine adenomas can occur throughout the small intestine; even in patients with no colonic polyps and no history of familial adenomatous polyposis (FAP). They occur more frequently in the duodenum than in the jejunum, and more frequently in the jejunum than in the ileum. They are sometimes multiple. They may complicate Crohn's disease and can be observed in ileostomies as a late complication following surgery for ulcerative colitis.[20]

Macroscopic appearance

- Adenomas are usually pedunculated.

- The stalk can be several centimetres long, leaving the polyp free to move back and forth in a segment.

- The surface is usually lobulated and red in colour (Fig 4.10).

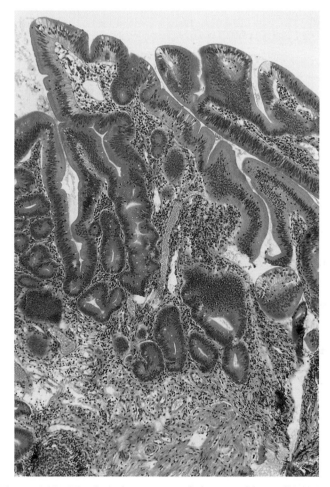

Figure 4.11 – Histological appearance of adenoma of the small intestine, note the close similarity to colonic adenoma.

Microscopic features

Similar to colonic adenomas (see p. 110 in Chapter 5).

Biological behaviour and associated conditions

There is evidence that points to an adenoma–carcinoma sequence similar to that found in the colon, although small intestinal lesions have been less well studied.[21]

Presenting symptoms are non-specific and include gastro-intestinal bleeding, anaemia, abdominal pain and partial intestinal obstruction or intussusception.[22]

Management

Endoscopic or surgical resection should be considered if the lesion is large or inducing symptoms.

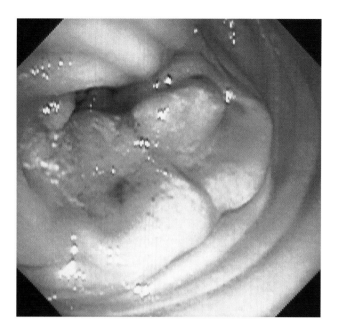

Figure 4.12 – Small intestinal adenocarcinoma is usually a large, nodular and ulcerated lesion. A polypoid appearance is rare.

ADENOCARCINOMA

Prevalence

Adenocarcinoma of the jejunum or ileum is a rare primary neoplasm. Most tumours occur in patients aged between 50 and 70 years. Approximately one-third of small intestinal adenocarcinoma found in the jejunum and ileum.

Most jejunal adenocarcinoma occurs within the first 30 cm from the ligament of Treitz.[23]

Endoscopic appearance

- Usually single, occasionally multifocal (Fig 4.12).

- Approximately one-fifth of the tumours are polypoid; the remaining four-fifths are annular lesions.[24]

Microscopic features

Similar to their colonic counterparts (see p. 114 in Chapter 5 and Fig 4.13).

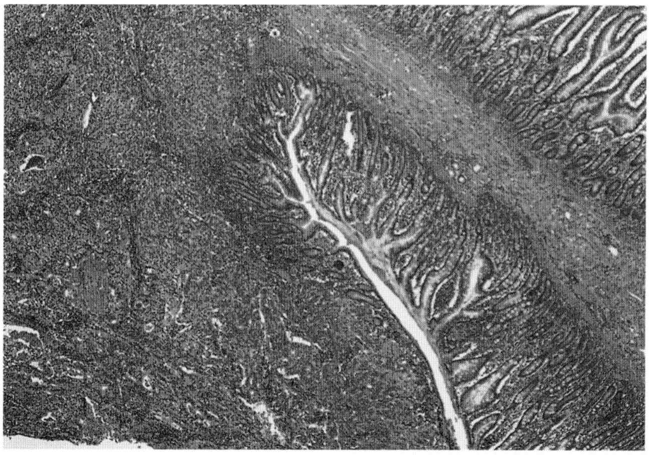

Figure 4.13 – Microscopic examination shows a moderately differentiated adenocarcinoma, which is deeply invasive, and the transition with normal intestinal mucosa.

Biological behaviour and associated conditions

The five-year survival rate is approximately 30%.[24] Gastrointestinal bleeding, obstruction and systemic symptoms (such as weight loss, anorexia, crampy abdominal pain, nausea, vomiting and fever) are frequently noted.

There is evidence for an association between small bowel adenocarcinoma and Crohn's enterocolitis and coeliac disease.

Patients with Crohn's disease who develop carcinoma do so 10–20 years earlier than those without Crohn's. In Crohn's disease more multifocal carcinomas are found. Carcinomas occur more commonly in the ileum.[25]

Management

Surgical resection, which can be followed by adjuvant therapy depending on the staging of the lesion.

METASTATIC TUMOURS

Synonyms

Secondary deposits.

Prevalence

In a series of 4101 necropsy cases with various primary malignancies small intestinal metastases were found in 3.8% of the patients.[26]

Macroscopic appearance

- Haematogenous spread of the tumour to the small intestine occurs most commonly in patients with carcinoma of the lung, breast (especially lobular carcinoma) or melanoma. These nodular lesions tend to occur on the anti-mesenteric border.

- Metastases in the small intestine are most often multiple and present as intramural masses. They bulge into the lumen and produce sessile or pedunculated polypoid structures (Fig 4.14).

- Although predominantly submucosal growths, a common appearance is an elevated mucosal plaque that shows central ulceration.

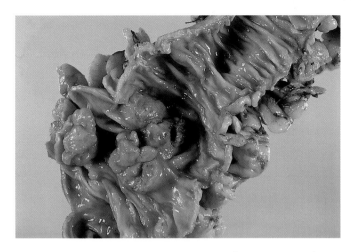

Figure 4.14 – Macroscopic appearance of metastatic malignant melanoma appearing as polypoidal nodules that are sometimes difficult to differentiate from primary polypoidal nodules, except that they are usually multiple and present as intraluminal masses.

Microscopic features

Secondary carcinomas may not involve the mucosa. They characteristically lack a component of adenoma or severe dysplasia in the margin of the tumour (Figs 4.15 & 4.16). The histological diagnosis can be difficult (if the primary tumour is unknown) and immunohistochemistry may be needed.[27] This is particularly true in cases of metastatic malignant melanomas.

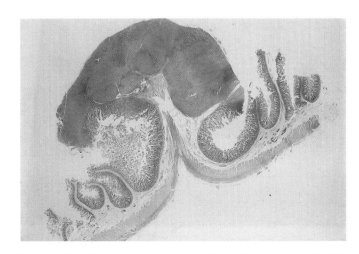

Figure 4.15 – A whole mount of one of the nodules shown in Fig 4.14.

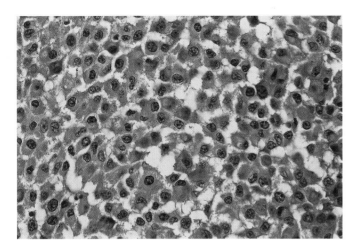

Figure 4.16 – A higher power of the malignant melanoma lesion in Fig 4.15 showing the typical cellular features of the tumour.

Biological behaviour and associated conditions

Metastases to the small bowel most frequently manifest as an obstruction. Perforation or haemorrhage may also occur. Often they are incidental findings at autopsy.

Management

In symptomatic cases palliative surgery should be performed. Adjuvant chemotherapy could be considered in selected cases depending upon the nature of the primary tumour.

ENDOCRINE TUMOURS

Synonyms

Terminology is a source of confusion. The term carcinoid is commonly considered to be interchangeable with 'neuro-endocrine tumour'. In actual fact, a carcinoid is a serotonin-producing endocrine tumour with defined clinical features. The term carcinoid has also been used for well differentiated neuroendocrine tumours.

Prevalence

Unlike carcinomas, carcinoid tumours are more common in the ileum. Most tumours occur in patients aged between 50 and 70 years.[28,29]

Atypical carcinoids, neuroendocrine carcinomas and adeno-carcinoids are uncommon in the small bowel.

Macroscopic appearance

- Ileal endocrine tumours are usually either sessile, umbilicated nodules or ulcerated tumours.

- Less commonly they protrude into the lumen as a polyp.

- The cut surface is yellowish in colour and the tumour is located either in the submucosa or deeper (Fig 4.17).

- Approximately 30% of ileal endocrine tumours are multiple (Fig 4.18).

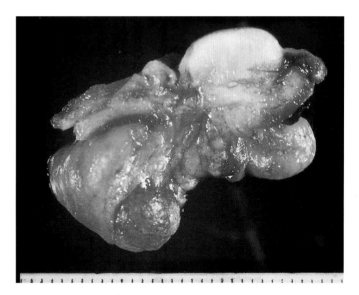

Figure 4.17 – Surgical specimen showing the presence of multiple small carcinoid nodules, one of them with yellow cut surface.

Microscopic features

The tumour consists of small regular cells that grow in nests, trabecula, cords, tubules, or sheets and may form rosettes (Figs 4.19 & 4.20). Mitoses and cellular pleomorphism are rare.

Classic endocrine tumours stain positively with argyrophil and argentaffin stains and are also positive for chromo-granin. Immunohistochemical studies have localized sero-tonin, substance P and other substances in these tumours.

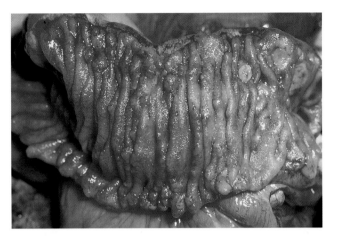

Figure 4.18 – Surgical specimen of ileum revealing multiple carcinoid tumours which appear polypoid.

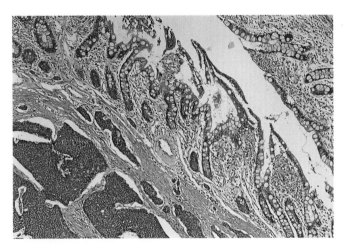

Figure 4.19 – Low power magnification of an endocrine tumour. Note the neoplastic cells are arranged in compartments separated by thick fibrous tissue.

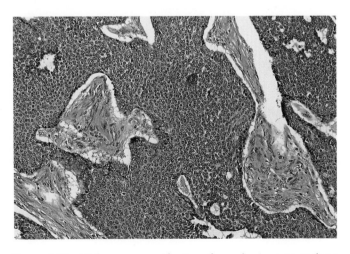

Figure 4.20 – High power magnification of an endocrine tumour showing solid nests of neoplastic cells with a monotonous appearance and peripheral palisading.

Biological behaviour and associated conditions

Carcinoids may *either* manifest as small bowel obstruction, metastases, bowel ischaemia or part of multiple endocrine syndrome (MEN), *or* they may be found incidentally.

Carcinoid tumours have been reported to occur in association with a variety of other neoplasms (in the stomach, colon, etc) and inflammatory diseases (inflammatory bowel disease and coeliac disease).

Management

Surgical resection is the treatment of choice. Adjuvant chemotherapy can be considered.

HAEMANGIOMAS

Synonyms

Benign vascular tumours.

Prevalence

Intestinal haemangiomas account for about 10% of all benign intestinal tumours and occur predominantly in the jejunum.[30] The majority are solitary, localized lesions.

Endoscopic appearance

- At endoscopy they appear as small, soft, blue-red, mucosal nodules or intraluminal polyps (Fig 4.21).

- The polypoid type of cavernous haemangioma is as frequent as the infiltrating type.[31]

Microscopic features

Histologically they consist of irregularly-sized vascular channels (Fig 4.22). Three main types are considered: cavernous, capillary and mixed haemangiomas.

They must be distinguished from telangiectasias of Rendu–Osler's disease, arteriovenous malformations, Kaposi's sarcoma and angiodysplasia.

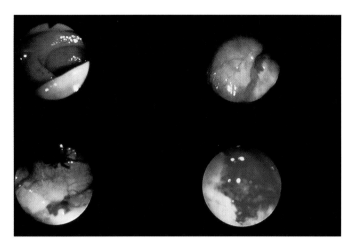

Figure 4.21 – Endoscopic appearance of haemangioma.

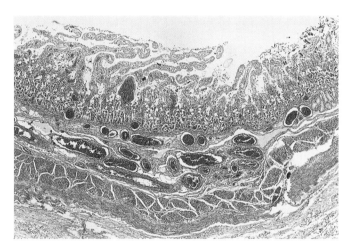

Figure 4.22 – Microphotograph of small intestine biopsy of a case of haemangioma showing the presence in the submucosa of a complex of irregular dilated vessels.

Arteriovenous malformations, occurring in patients younger than 50 years, may occasionally be seen.[32]

Biological behaviour and associated conditions

Symptoms are mainly gastrointestinal bleeding or anaemia.

Management

Patients with solitary haemangioma do not need to be followed up. For bleeding lesions a surgical treatment is usually indicated. Endoscopic haemostasis may be performed if the lesion is accessible by, for example, an enteroscope.[33]

KAPOSI'S SARCOMA

Prevalence

Multi-system neoplastic disease, which is uncommon in mild climates but endemic in tropical Africa, and on which attention has been focused since Acquired Immune Deficiency Syndrome (AIDS) dramatically increased in prevalence.

The gastrointestinal tract is the most common site of visceral involvement with the small intestine being the most frequently affected area.[26,34]

Endoscopic appearance

- The disease may appear as submucosal, mulberry-like, red-violaceous nodules that often occur as multiple lesions with endoscopic features such as macro-papular lesions of 5 mm or more with minimal elevation (Fig 4.23).

- The disease can also appear as irregular polypoid lesions of variable size, ranging from 5–10 mm and sometimes as umbilicated nodules that are 10 mm or more in diameter.

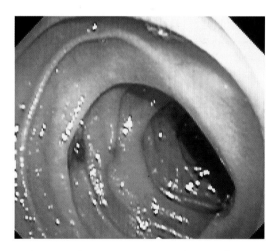

Figure 4.23 – Kaposi's sarcoma appears endoscopically as small, red-violaceous nodules, as in this small intestinal location.

Microscopic features

The tumour is composed of vascular structures lined by pleomorphic endothelial cells that show nuclear atypia with a high mitotic activity and a population of atypical stromal spindle cells also with nuclear atypia (Fig 4.24).

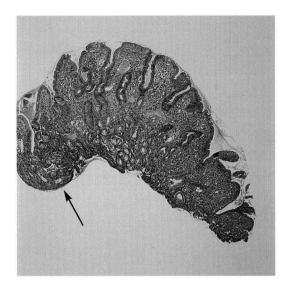

A

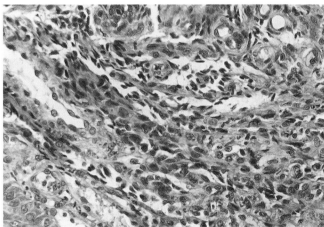

B

Figure 4.24 – (a) Photomicrograph of a small intestinal endoscopic biopsy showing an irregular vascular proliferation as seen at the edge of a Kaposi's sarcoma. (b) High power view of (a) showing proliferation of vascular channels, lined in some places by plump endothelial cells.

Biological behaviour and associated conditions

Kaposi's sarcoma is associated with immune deficiency conditions, such as AIDS and post-transplantation state. Usually this is clinically silent but complications such as bleeding, intussusception, perforation and protein loss can occur.

Management

Surgery, radiotherapy and anti-neoplastic agents can result in some improvement.

LYMPHANGIOMAS

Synonyms and related terms

Cystic lymphangiomas, cystic hygromas.

Prevalence

These are rare lesions that can occur at any age in adult life. Lymphangioma must be distinguished from the more common simple lymphatic cysts that appear as small (1–2 cm), submucosal, yellow nodules.[35] Lymphatic cysts are also called chylangioma or chylous (lymphangiectatic) cysts. They neither produce symptoms nor cause protein loss.

Endoscopic appearance

- Lymphangiomas may present *either* as small, single or multiple mucosal polyps *or* as large intramural masses.

- They are soft, pink or yellow circumscribed lesions.

Microscopic features

Unilocular or multilocular cysts composed of vascular channels lined by flattened endothelial cells in a loose myxoid stroma (Fig 4.25).

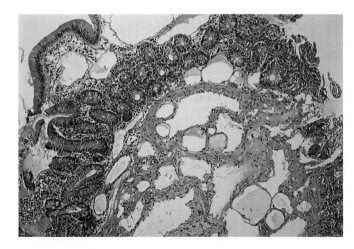

Figure 4.25 – This shows a case of lymphangioma that can be characterized by the presence of dilated thin-walled lymphatics in the mucosa, submucosa or both, as seen in this case. Most small intestinal lymphangiomas appear as small, soft yellow, slightly elevated lesions.

Biological behaviour and associated conditions

Usually asymptomatic.

Management

No follow-up is needed.

STROMAL TUMOURS OF THE SMALL INTESTINE

Mesenchymal tumours of the small bowel include those of smooth muscle, adipose, vascular and neural tissue origin as well as a group of tumours of indeterminate origin. Because it is often difficult to classify some of these tumours on routinely stained slides, the term 'Gastrointestinal Stromal Tumour' (GIST) has been proposed. Immunohisto-chemistry is now commonly used for the identification of these tumours (c-kit or CD117 positive or negative).

LEIOMYOMA – LEIOMYOSARCOMA

Synonyms

Smooth muscle tumours.

Prevalence

In the small intestine benign stromal tumours with smooth muscle differentiation (leiomyomas) are rare compared with other segments of the gastrointestinal tract. Nevertheless, they are one of the most common benign tumours of the small bowel. They occur throughout the small bowel with almost equal frequency in the jejunum and ileum.

Leiomyosarcomas are the most frequent malignant soft tissue tumour of the small intestine.[36]

Macroscopic appearance

- Leiomyomas that originate in the submucosa appear as smooth, oval or round and are occasionally pedunculated (Figs 4.26–4.28).

- Leiomyosarcomas are usually large necrotic tumours and not really polypoid.

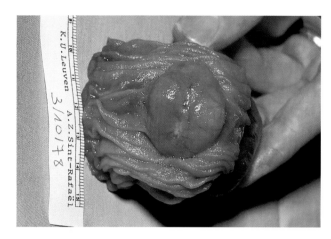

Figure 4.26 – Surgical specimen of a small intestinal benign smooth muscle tumour.

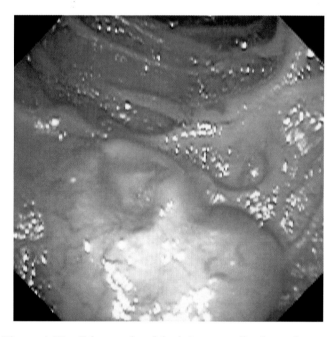

Figure 4.27 – Submucosal nodular lesion, centrally ulcerated, corresponding histologically to a benign stromal tumour with smooth muscle differentiation.

Microscopic features

Almost all stromal tumours of the small bowel are composed of spindle cells.

In leiomyomas, the spindle cells tend to be organized in short fascicles that can be separated by fine fibrovascular septa (Fig 4.29). They may show palisading. In the deeper

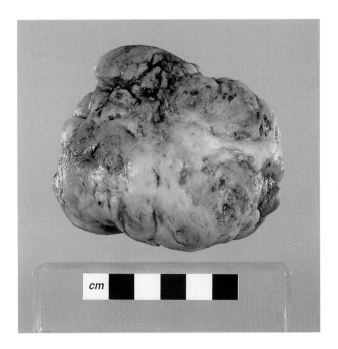

Figure 4.28 – Solitary leiomyoma removed from a small intestine.

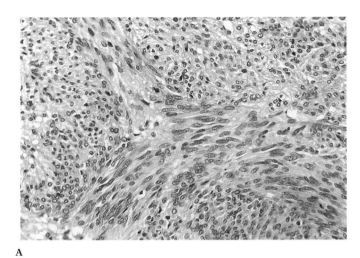

A

B

Figure 4.29 – Histological appearance of smooth muscle tumour showing a typical aspect of leiomyoma as seen on routine haematoxylin and eosin stain and (*b*) immunohistochemistry using antibodies against alpha smooth muscle actin.

part of the lesion, dense hyaline balls composed of normal collagen fibres may be found. Mitoses are infrequent.

Features that indicate malignancy are: a high number of mitoses (counts in excess of 10 per 50 high-power fields), increased cellularity, necrosis and large tumour size (over 5 cm).

Biological behaviour and associated conditions

Leiomyomas are often asymptomatic. Gastrointestinal bleeding in a young to middle-aged adult is the most likely clinical presentation. Pedunculated lesions may cause intussusception.

Leiomyosarcomas may cause bleeding, obstruction, pain or may even perforate.[37]

Management

Treatment is usually surgical. Follow-up is indicated for tumours with features of malignancy.

NEUROGENIC POLYPS

Synonyms and related terms

Schwannoma, neurilemmoma, neurofibroma, neurinoma, ganglioneuroma.

Prevalence

These are exceedingly rare tumours.

Many of the cases reported in the literature are in fact identical to those reported as smooth muscle tumours or GISTs.

Neurofibroma and neurofibromatosis occur more commonly in the small intestine, while ganglioneuromas appear to be largely centred in the colon.[38]

Isolated neurofibromas occur most commonly in the ileum whereas the jejunum is involved in von Recklinghausen's disease.[39]

Macroscopic appearance

- They present rarely as intraluminal masses.
- Neurofibromas can occur as round or oval masses.

Microscopic features

Neurilemmoma is usually an encapsulated tumour showing palisading of nuclei. The nuclei tend to be thin and wavy (Figs 4.30 & 4.31). Demonstration of S100 protein can help to confirm the diagnosis.

Neurofibromas are irregular proliferations of enteroglial cells, neurites and fibroblasts.

Biological behaviour and associated conditions

Neurofibromas are usually seen in von Recklinghausen's disease.

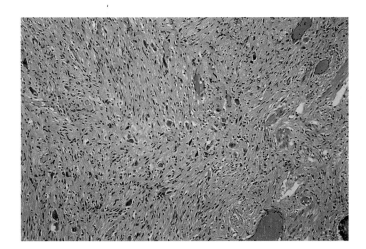

Figure 4.30 – Low power magnification of a case with ganglioneuroma. Note the large ganglion cells are distributed amongst spindle cell neural tissue.

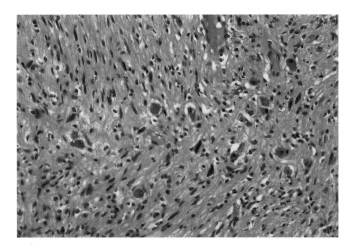

Figure 4.31 – This is a higher magnification of the lesion shown in Fig 4.30 in which the ganglion cells with peripherally situated nuclei are well illustrated.

Management

Surgery is the treatment of choice in cases of ganglioneuromatosis and even with isolated neurofibroma.

Long-term follow-up is required because of the possible association with von Recklinghausen's disease or multiple endocrine neoplastic syndrome type IIb (medullary carcinoma of the thyroid, adrenal pheochromocytoma, mucosal neuromas and skeletal abnormalities).

GUT AUTONOMIC NERVE TUMOURS (GANT) POLYP

Synonyms

Plexosarcomas, subset of GISTs.

Prevalence

These are rare tumours, with fewer than fifty cases published up to 2000. They occur more commonly in the small intestine and arise from autonomic nervous plexuses (Meissner, Auerbach).[40,41]

Macroscopic appearance

- Large, multilobular, circumscribed tumours which may have a polypoidal configuration.

Microscopic features

Composed of characteristic spindle cells, resembling the typical spindle cell smooth muscle tumour (Figs 4.32 & 4.33).

Ultrastructural and immunohistochemical analysis is needed for precise identification.

Biological behaviour and associated conditions

Malignant, metastasising tumour. Many patients reported thus far did not survive for more than 9–10 months.

Transperitoneal spread is a charateristic feature.

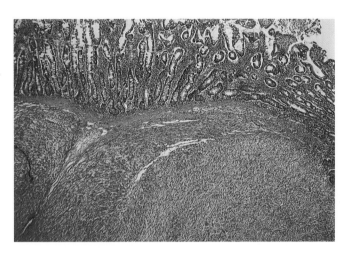

Figure 4.32 – Microscopic picture of a GANT tumour of the small intestine. The mucosa is still largely intact and covers a tumour composed of numerous interlacing bundles.

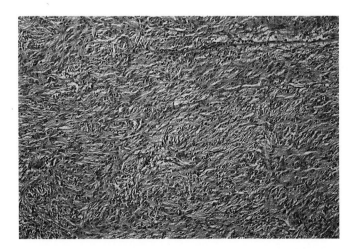

Figure 4.33 – Higher power magnification of GANT. Note the spindle cell proliferation of the tumour that on routine stains appears to be similar to that in smooth muscle tumours or GISTs.

Management

Surgical resection.

GRANULAR CELL TUMOURS

Synonyms

Granular cell myoblastomas.

Prevalence

Exceedingly rare in the small intestine.[42]

Macroscopic appearance

- As elsewhere in the gastrointestinal tract, they are small yellow or white intramural masses or plaques.[43]
- They usually measure 1–4 cm.

Microscopic features

Similar to those seen in other areas of the gastrointestinal tract. (See also p. 15 in Chapter 1).

Biological behaviour

Usually benign.

LIPOMAS

Related terms

Angiolipomas (when abundant vascular channels are present).

Fibrolipomas (when scattered collagen bands are present).

Atypical lipomas (when adipocyte atypia is present).

Prevalence

Lipomas of the small intestine are rare. In a recent review, only 73 cases of jejunal and 111 ileal lipomas had been reported.[26]

Macroscopic appearance

- They are generally solitary, well circumscribed, smooth, round, soft, intramural white or yellow masses (Fig 4.34). They are occasionally ulcerated.

- Multiple lipomas have been described in middle-aged to elderly patients.[44]

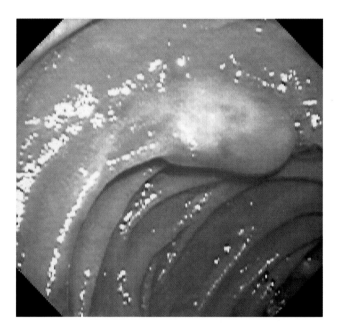

Figure 4.34 – Small intestinal lipomas are usually solitary, well circumscribed, soft, yellow or white lesions.

Microscopic features

Lipomas are composed of uniform adipose cells (Fig. 4.35). They may compress the muscularis mucosae and often cause thinning of the overlying mucosa.

Larger tumours can undergo necrosis which may be followed by the formation of lipogranulomas.

Occasionally, the adipose tissue can be mixed with more or less abundant fibrous septae and vessels.

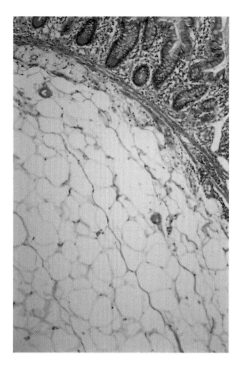

Figure 4.35 – Low power photograph of a lipoma partially covered by small intestinal mucosa.

Biological behaviour and associated conditions

They are benign lesions. Symptoms are not present in the majority of cases, however bleeding and intussusception may occur. They are not known to be associated with other conditions.

Lipomatosis of the caecal valve should be distinguished from true lipoma.

Management

Resection, either surgically or endoscopically, is recommended for symptomatic lesions.

LYMPHOID POLYP

Synonyms and related terms

Focal lymphoid hyperplasia, nodular lymphoid hyperplasia.

Prevalence

This is a rare lesion.

Endoscopic appearance

- Lymphoid hyperplasia presents as a nodular or polypoid lesion and can be up to 0.5 cm in diameter. It may be single or multiple. The latter is more common in the ileum.[45]

Microscopic features

They are characterized by the presence of hyperplastic lymphoid follicles, with enlarged germinal centres accompanied by villous distortions (Fig 4.36).

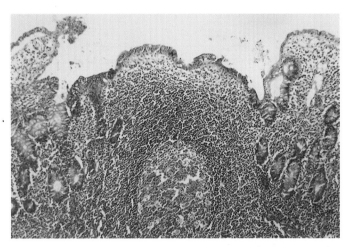

Figure 4.36 – Microscopic appearance of lymphoid polyp, in which lymphoid follicles are seen, sometimes with germinal centres.

Biological behaviour and associated conditions

Diffuse nodular lymphoid hyperplasia complicates some adult forms of hypogammaglobulinaemia.[46] (See also p. 61 in Chapter 3.)

Must be differentiated from lymphoma, especially malignant lymphomatous polyposis.

Management

No specific treatment is needed for lymphoid polyps, but if the lesion occurs as part of the disease spectrum of hypo-

gammaglobulinaemia then the underlying disease should be treated.

LYMPHOMAS

Synonyms

Malignant lymphomas.

Prevalence

The gastrointestinal tract is the commonest location of extranodal non-Hodgkin's lymphoma.

The small intestine is the second most frequent site (30%) after the stomach. Malignant lymphomas make up about 20% of all malignant tumours that occur in the small bowel.

Most lymphomas occur in the distal small intestine, except in patients with malabsorption (coeliac disease) when proximal sites predominate.

Macroscopic appearance

- The gross presentation is variable.
- In 10–20% of patients, multiple small bowel lesions are found.
- Irrespective of the histological type, small intestinal lymphomas may take any of the following forms:
  - multiple nodules
  - an infiltrating tumour
  - a polypoid mass (Fig 4.37)
  - an endophytic mass with excavation and fistula formation.[47]

Microscopic features

Various types of lymphomas can affect the small intestine. At present there is no single classification that is regarded as entirely satisfactory. Morphological, immunological, cyto-

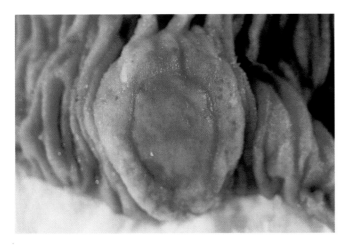

Figure 4.37 – A case of polypoid lymphoma of the small bowel.

genetic and molecular biological techniques are currently used for a proper diagnosis.[48,49]

The small intestine is affected by: (1) mantle cell lymphoma, a B-cell lymphoma of small to medium-sized cells, usually showing a diffuse growth pattern, presenting as a malignant lymphomatous polyposis; (2) low grade B-cell lymphoma of mucosa-associated lymphoid tissue (extranodal marginal zone B-cell lymphoma) composed of small lymphocytes showing a diffuse growth pattern; (3) diffuse large B-cell lymphoma with large cells having a prominent nucleolus (Fig 4.38); (4) Burkitt's lymphoma, composed of monomorphic medium-sized cells and showing a starry sky pattern due to macrophages, affecting the ileum in particular; (5) intestinal T-cell lymphoma (with or without enteropathy) composed of small, medium or large anaplastic cells, but which presents rarely in a polypoid form.

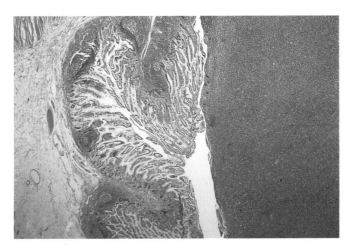

Figure 4.38 – Photomicrograph of a case of lymphoma.

Biological behaviour and associated conditions

The majority of patients are symptomatic (weight loss, diarrhoea, perforation).

The prognosis depends not only upon the type of lymphoma but also on the extent of the disease.

Lymphomas can be:

- curable if localized (low grade B-cell lymphoma of Mucosa-Associated Lymphoid Tissue (MALT));

- aggressive but potentially curable (diffuse large B-cell lymphoma);

- moderately aggressive (and not usually curable) with a mean survival of 3–5 years (lymphomatous polyposis);

- aggressive (intestinal T-cell lymphoma)

- highly aggressive (Burkitt's lymphoma).

Management

Surgery, with or without chemotherapy, for curative or palliative treatment are the options.[50]

REFERENCES

1. Segal GH, Petras RE: Small intestine. In *Histology for Pathologists*, Sternberg S (ed.). New York, Raven Press 1992: pp. 547–572

2. Yamamoto T: Jejunum and villi: structural basis of intestinal absorption. In *Ultrastructure of the Digestive Tract*, Motta PM, Fujita H (eds). Boston, Martinus Nijhoff Publishing 1988: pp. 85–99

3. Lee SM, Mosenthal WT, Weismann RE: Tumorous heterotopic gastric mucosa in the small intestine. *Arch Surg* 1970; **100:** 619–622

4. Barbosa JJ, Dockerty MB, Waugh JM: Pancreatic heterotopia. *Surg Gynecol Obstet* 1946; **82:** 527–542

5. Soule EH, Hallenbeck GA: Polypoid gastric heterotopia of the jejunum and ileum causing subacute intestinal obstruction. *Surg Gynecol Obstet* 1959; **108:** 282–288

6. Schutter FW, Kimm K, Kiroff P: Dystoper magenpolyp als Ursacher der Invagination eines Meckel'schen Divertikels. *Chirurg* 1995; **66:** 1016–1018

7. Morson B: Some peculiarities in the histology of intestinal polyps. *Dis Colon Rectum* 1972; **5:** 337–344

8. Bracke PG, Degryse HR, Goovaerts GC, *et al*: Polypoid hamartoma of the jejunum. *Gastrointest Radiol* 1991; **16:** 113–114

9. Mazzeo S, De Liperi A, Sbragia P et al: Diagnostica per imagini delle invaginazioni intestinali dell'adulto. Descrizione di 9 casi. Radiol Med Torino 1995; **90:** 49–55

10. Hizawa K, Sida M, Matsumoto T, et al: Neoplastic transformation arising in Peutz–Jeghers polyposis. Dis Colon Rectum 1993; **36:** 953–957

11. Rossini FP, Arrigoni A, Pennazio M: Clinical Enteroscopy. J Clin Gastroenterol 1996; **22:** 231–235

12. Harned RK, Buck JL, Shekitka KM: Inflammatory fibroid polyps of the gastrointestinal tract: radiologic evaluation. Radiology 1992; **182:** 863–866

13. Williams GR, Jaffe S, Scott CA: Inflammatory fibroid polyp of the terminal ileum presenting in a patient with active Crohn's disease. Histopathology 1992; **20:** 545–547

14. Widgren S, Pizzolato GP: Inflammatory fibroid polyp of the gastrointestinal tract: possible origin in myofibroblast? A study of twelve cases. Ann Pathol 1987; **7:** 183–192

15. Shimer GR, Helwig EB: Inflammatory fibroid polyps of the intestine. Am J Clin Pathol 1984; **81:** 708–714

16. De Foer B, Serrien B, Bleus E, et al: Inflammatory fibroid polyp of the ileum. Abdom Imaging 1993; **18:** 363–365

17. Allibone RO, Hoffman J, Gosney JR, Helliwell TR: Granulation tissue polyposis associated with carcinoid tumours of the small intestine. Histopathology 1993; **22:** 475–480

18. Kahn E, Daum F: Pseudopolyps of the small intestine in Crohn's disease. Hum Pathol 1984; **15:** 84–86

19. Vantrappen G, Geboes K: Yersinia enterocolitica. In Diarrhées aiguës infectieuses, Rambaud JC, Rampal P (eds). Paris, Doin Éditeurs 1993: pp. 101–112

20. Gourtsoyiannis NC, Bays D, Papaioannou N, et al: Benign tumors of the small intestine: preoperative evaluation with a barium infusion technique. Eur J Radiol 1993; **16:** 115–125

21. Suarez V, Alexander-Williams J, O'Connor HJ, et al: Carcinoma developing in ileostomies after 25 or more years. Gastroenterology 1988; **95:** 205–208

22. Pennazio M, Arrigoni A, Risio M, et al: Clinical evaluation of push type enteroscopy. Endoscopy 1995; **27:** 164–170

23. Herbsman H, Wetstein L, Rosen Y, et al: Tumours of the small intestine. Curr Probl Surg 1980; **17:** 126–183

24. Bridge MF, Perzin KH: Primary adenocarcinoma of the jejunum and ileum. A clinicopathologic study. Cancer 1975; **36:** 1876–1887

25. Fresko D, Lazarus SS, Dotan J, Reingold M: Early presentation of carcinoma of the small bowel in Crohn's disease ('Crohn's carcinoma'). Gastroenterology 1982; **82:** 783–789

26. Widgren S: Rare and secondary (metastatic) tumours. In Gastrointestinal and Oesophageal Pathology, 2nd edn, Whitehead R (ed.). Edinburgh, Churchill-Livingstone 1995: pp. 849–861

27. Nariat T, Nakazawa H, Hizawa Y, et al: Hepatocellular carcinoma with unusual metastasis to the small intestine. Acta Pathol Japan 1993; **43:** 779–782

28. North JH, Pack MS: Malignant tumours of small intestine. Ann Surg 2000; **66:** 46–51

29. Moertel CG, Sauer G, Dockcrty MB, Baggenstoss AH: Life history of the carcinoid tumour of the small intestine. Cancer 1961; **14:** 901–912

30. Camilleri M, Chadwick VS, Hodgson HJF: Vascular anomalies of the gastrointestinal tract. Hepatogastroenterology 1984; **31:** 149–153

31. Jass JR: Tumors of the small and large intestines (including the anal region). In Diagnostic Histopathology of Tumors. Fletcher CDM (ed.). Edinburgh, Churchill Livingstone 1995: pp. 243–254

32. Guarner J, Grossman B, Judd R, et al: Multiple arteriovenous malformations of the small intestine in a patient with protein S deficiency. Am J Clin Pathol 1989; **92:** 374–378

33. Frinberger E, Hagenmuller F, Classen M: Endostomy: a new approach to small bowel endoscopy. Endoscopy 1989; **21:** 86–88

34. Port JH, Traube J, Winans S: The visceral manifestations of Kaposi's sarcoma. Gastrointest Endosc 1982; **28:** 179–181

35. Aase S, Gundersen R: Submucous lymphatic cysts of the small intestine. Acta Pathol Microbiol Immunol Scand (A) 1983; **91:** 191–194

36. Ojha A, Zachert J, Scheuba C, et al: Primary small bowel malignancies. J Clin Gastroenterol 2000; **30:** 289–293

37. Wilson JM, Melvin DB, Gray GF, Thorbjarnarson B: Primary malignancies of the small bowel. Ann Surg 1974; **180:** 175–179

38. Shekitka KM, Sobin LH: Ganglioneuroma of the gastrointestinal tract. Relation to Von Recklinghausen disease and other multiple tumour syndromes. Am J Surg Pathol 1984; **18:** 250–257

39. Bruneton JN, Drouillard J, Roux P, et al: Les tumeurs nerveuses de l'intestin grêle. Revue de la littérature à propos de 6 cas personnels. Ann Gastroenterol Hepatol 1984; **20:** 79–84

40. Herrera GA, Cerezo L, Jones JE, et al: Gastrointestinal autonomic nerve tumours 'plexosarcomas'. Arch Pathol Lab Med 1989; **113:** 846–853

41. Drews G, Kiene S, Emmrich P, Lehmann J: Maligner Tumor des autonomen Nervensystems des Magens (GAN-Tumor) – Ein Fallbericht einer neuen Entitdt. Zent bl Chir 1992; **117:** 564–568

42. Johnston J, Helwig EB: Granular cell tumours of the gastrointestinal tract and perianal region. A study of 74 cases. Dig Dis Sci 1981; **26:** 807–816

43. Gastrointestinal mesenchymal neoplasms. In Gastrointestinal Pathology; An Atlas and Text, 2nd edn, Fenoglio-Preiser CM, Noffsinger A, Stemmermann GN, Lantz P, Listrom MB, Rilke FO (eds). Philadelphia, New York, Lippincott-Raven 1998: **25:** pp. 1169–1315

44. Climie ARW, Wylin RF: Small intestinal lipomatosis. Arch Pathol Lab Med 1981; **105:** 40–42

45. Molas G, Potet F, Nogig P: Hyperplasie lymphoide focale (pseudolymphome) de l'ileon terminal chez l'adulte. Gastroenterol Clin Biol 1985; **9:** 630–633

46. Van den Brande P, Geboes K, Vantrappen G, et al: Intestinal nodular lymphoid hyperplasia in patients with common variable immunodeficiency: local accumulation of B and CD8(+) lymphocytes. J Clin Immunol 1988; **8:** 296–306

47. Marshak RH, Lindner AE, Maklansky D: Lymphoreticular disorders of the gastrointestinal tract. *Gastrointest Radiol* 1979; **4:** 103–120

48. Chan JKC, Banks PM, Cleary ML, *et al*: A revised European–American classification of lymphoid neoplasms proposed by the International Lymphoma Study Group. *Am J Clin Pathol* 1995; **103:** 543–560

49. O'Briain DS, Kennedy MJ, Daly PA, *et al*: Multiple lymphomatous polyposis of the gastrointestinal tract. A clinicopathologically distinctive form of non-Hodgkin's lymphoma of B-cell centrocytic type. *Am J Surg Pathol* 1989; **13:** 691–699

50. Jaser N, Sivula A: Primary small intestinal non-Hodgkin's lymphoma in Finland 1972–1977. Clinical presentation and results of treatment. *Ann Chir Gynaecol* 1991; **80:** 250–257

Polyps of the Large Intestine

N A Shepherd

INTRODUCTION

Polyps of the large intestine are very common and represent a considerable proportion of the practising endoscopist's and pathologist's workload. Although the term polyp has been defined previously in this volume, it is important to reaffirm that a polyp is any lesion raised above an epithelial surface. In our experience many practitioners continue to equate the word polyp with adenoma and this may have serious implications for patient management, particularly if the polyps are multiple. There are many types of large intestinal polyp and the different types show considerable variation in their presentation, morphological appearance, clinical significance and neoplastic risk. This emphasises the importance of sound histological assessment to ensure an accurate diagnosis and appropriate management of patients. Most of these polyp types also have a parallel polyposis syndrome (see Chapter 6). Nevertheless it is important to note that large intestinal polyps are often, indeed usually, multiple and this is one of the reasons behind the difficulties in definition of some of the polyposis syndromes.

Polyps of the large intestine can originate from both mucosal and submucosal tissues. Hyperplastic and neoplastic conditions of other tissues within and without the bowel wall can also present as polyps, although these are not usually considered in standard polyp classifications. It is evident that any polyp demands histopathological assessment to confirm its true nature, that there is no complication such as malignancy in an adenoma and, in certain situations, that it is completely excised. Polyps resected at endoscopy do comprise a significant workload in the average histopathology laboratory and consistently provide diagnostic problems.

NORMAL STRUCTURE

Surgical anatomy

The large intestine comprises the appendix, caecum, colon and rectum. It measures about 150 cm long from the pole of the caecum to the dentate line, at the junction of the rectum and the anus. The appendix measures only between 0.5 and 1.0 cm in diameter and is between 4 and 11 cm long. It arises from the pole of the caecum and may take up one of three positions – anterior to the caecum, below the caecum and retrocaecal. The colon's diameter steadily diminishes from proximal to distal apart from a dilatation in the rectum, known as the ampulla. Its physiological diameter is between 3.5 cm and 5 cm in the adult. The caecum is that part of the large intestine below a line from the centre of the ileo-caecal valve horizontally, laterally to the opposite aspect of the bowel. The remaining colon is divided into an ascending part (between the aforementioned line and the hepatic flexure), a transverse part (between the hepatic and splenic flexures), a descending part (between the splenic flexure and the point where the colon crosses the pelvic brim) and a sigmoid part (which ends at the rectosigmoid junction). The hepatic and splenic flexures are those parts of the colon where it effectively turns around 90 degrees in a clockwise direction closely related to the liver and spleen, respectively.

The rectum measures 15 cm in length, approximately, and extends from the dentate line to the rectosigmoid junction. There are no absolutely definite anatomical landmarks on which the rectosigmoid junction can be defined. This accounts for the variations, in part, in the prevalence of sigmoid colonic and rectal cancers in different series. The rectum can be divided into three segments, the lower, middle and upper, each about 5 cm in length. Distinguishing between these three rectal segments is particularly important for the surgery and pathology of rectal cancer because of the differences in investment by the mesorectal tissues on the one hand and peritoneum on the other.

The colon and rectum are variably invested in peritoneum. The appendix is predominantly covered by peritoneum except for the mesoappendix and the caecum is completely invested. The ascending and descending colons are covered only on their anterior surfaces. Thus they are partly retroperitoneal structures. The transverse and sigmoid colon have well formed mesocolons and hence are invested by peritoneum completely apart from where they are attached to their respective mesocolons. The anterior peritoneal reflection, related to the rectum, is surprisingly low down and thus, in most patients, the anterior aspect of the upper rectum is completely invested by peritoneum. The reflection is highly variable in position but is notably lower in women, in whom it is usually only about 5–7 cm above the anorectal junction. The remainder of the rectum is surrounded by connective tissues, or mesorectum, which contains blood vessels, nerves and the haemorrhoidal or mesorectal lymph nodes. The mesorectum is contained within Denonvillier's fascia. These anatomical relationships are especially important for rectal cancer surgery, since it is now accepted that, for lower and middle rectal cancer at least, complete removal of the mesorectum can dramatically reduce local recurrence rates.

Histological features

The various parts of the large intestine have a similar histological structure, being composed of a relatively flat mucosa (Fig 5.1), submucosa containing connective tissues, muscularis propria and an adventitial or subserosal layer. The mucosa is not completely flat because it is thrown up into small hillocks, between small furrows, known as the innominate grooves (Fig 5.2). The muscularis propria has, like other parts of the gut, two layers, the inner circular and the outer longitudinal. The former is continuous and of a fairly consistent thickness whereas the longitudinal layer is also continuous but is concentrated in three bands, the taeniae coli, whose presence accounts for the longitudinal shortening of the colon resulting in the mucosal folds or plicae semilunares. Unlike the small bowel where the valvulae conniventes are circumferential, the plicae in the colon are gathered in three parallel lines between the taeniae.

The large intestine has a consistent histology throughout and the only variations at different sites of the bowel are in the amount of lymphoid tissue and lymphoglandular complexes and the epithelial cellular constituents. The mucosa is

composed of crypts arranged in parallel and lined by cells of the mucin-secreting and absorptive type. There are also specialised cells within the crypt, including neuroendocrine cells, Paneth cells and uncommitted stem cells, which are found in the proliferative zone at the base of the crypts. Paneth cells are only found, in the normal large intestine, in the appendix, caecum and colon proximal to the hepatic flexure. Lymphoid tissue is particularly prominent in the appendix, especially in children and young adults, whereas the rectum and anal canal also have a wealth of lymphoglandular complexes. The latter are specialised aggregates of lymphoid tissue that have a surface epithelium composed of M cells, which have a role in the transfer of luminal antigens to the underlying lymphoid tissue to allow antigen recognition and an appropriate immune response. These complexes account, in part, for the fine nodularity of the colorectal mucosa. They may become enlarged in pathological states and lead to polypoid excrescenses.

The epithelial crypts or tubules are embedded in a fine connective tissue known as the lamina propria. This contains small blood vessels, nerves and fibroblasts, some of the latter being of a specialised type and closely related to the epithelial crypts, the pericryptal myofibroblasts. The lamina propria also contains lymphocytes, plasma cells, histiocytes, eosinophils and mast cells in modest numbers. The lymphocytes and plasma cells are concentrated in the superficial third of the mucosa, in line with their role in the immune surveillance of luminal antigens. Very few polymorphs are seen in normal mucosa except within the lumina of blood

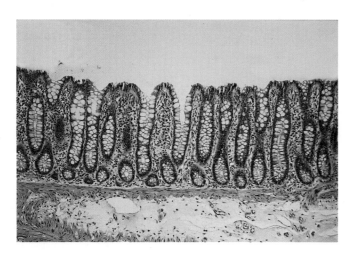

Figure 5.1 – The normal flat mucosa of the colorectum.

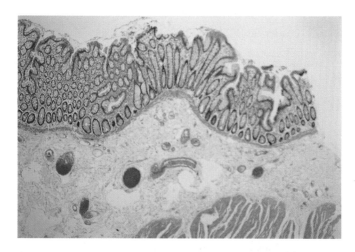

Figure 5.2 – Low power magnification of the rectal mucosa. Note the hillocks and the grooves of the large intestinal mucosa. This is a variation of the normal appearance.

vessels. Lymphatics are present in the deep mucosa and are particularly seen transecting the muscularis mucosae, the thin band of smooth muscle that separates the mucosa from the submucosa. However lymphatics do not extend up into the lamina propria.

JUVENILE POLYPS

Juvenile polyps are classified as hamartomas and consist of histologically normal tissues indigenous to the large intestine but arranged in a haphazard manner. It seems that the pathogenesis of the polyp is due to an excess of lamina propria. Recently it has been demonstrated that both sporadic juvenile polyps and those in the syndrome of juvenile polyposis share a molecular abnormality, which manifests itself in the fibroblasts of the lamina propria of the colorectal mucosa and not in the epithelium.[1] These data serve to re-affirm that these polyps are essentially a product of a molecular and histogenic abnormality of the lamina propria tissues.

Synonyms

Juvenile adenomas (this is a misnomer as there is no evidence of adenomatous change in solitary juvenile polyps in the great majority of cases).

Prevalence

Juvenile polyps are the commonest polyp in pre-adulthood years and are said to occur in about 1% of children.[2] Classical juvenile polyps are occasionally seen in adults.[3]

Juvenile polyps, in children and adults, are most commonly found in the rectum.

Endoscopic and gross appearance

- Although juvenile polyps are usually solitary and most usually demonstrated in the rectum, colonoscopic surveys have shown that they are on occasion multiple (any more than five should raise suspicions of juvenile polyposis (JP)) and evenly distributed throughout the colon.[3]

- They have a characteristic endoscopic appearance, being spherical and smooth: this latter is related to ulceration of the surface, which imparts a shiny red surface appearance to the polyp (Fig 5.3).

- Most polyps measure less than 10 mm in diameter but examples of polyps in excess of 2 cm have been recorded.

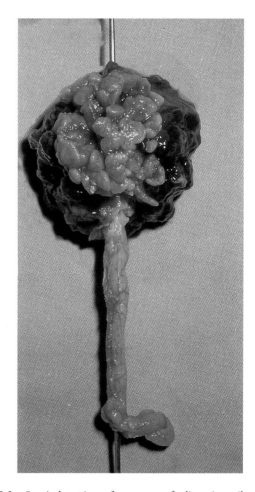

Figure 5.3 – Surgical specimen from a case of solitary juvenile polyp.

Microscopic features

The histological appearances of juvenile polyps are not entirely specific and polyps bearing a superficial resemblance to juvenile polyps are seen in inflammatory conditions (inflammatory polyps), at the site of ureterosigmoidostomy,[4] in Cowden's syndrome (see p. 140 in Chapter 6) and in various rarer syndromes.

The juvenile polyp is characterised by an abundant lamina propria: this seems to be the predominant pathogenetic factor in the development of the polyp, a view supported by molecular evidence concerning the molecular abnormality in both juvenile polyps and the corresponding polyposis, juvenile polyposis.[1]

This lamina propria lacks smooth muscle, in contrast to the other major 'hamartomatous' polyp of the intestines, the Peutz–Jeghers polyp, but occasionally there is stromal metaplasia to cartilage and/or bone.[5] Within the abundant lamina propria are irregularly branching, cystically dilated crypts lined, for the most part, by essentially normal colorectal-type epithelium (Fig 5.4). Metaplastic/hyperplastic foci are found in about 20% of juvenile polyps.[6] Surface ulceration is characteristic and accounts for the distinctive macroscopic appearances.

Biological behaviour and associated conditions

Juvenile polyps usually present with bleeding per rectum. Although sporadic polyps may be multiple, it is important to ensure that there is no evidence of juvenile polyposis, since this is a condition with considerable neoplastic potential (see p. 133 in Chapter 6).

Juvenile polyps themselves have a negligible neoplastic implication. There are only five reports, to our knowledge, documenting dysplastic change within sporadic juvenile polyps[6–11] and two cases describing carcinoma arising in solitary juvenile polyps.[12,13]

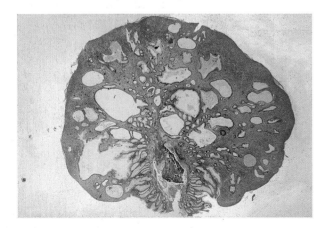

Figure 5.4 – Low power microphotograph of juvenile polyp showing an increase in the lamina propria, which lacks smooth muscle investing dilated crypts.

Management

Patients with a solitary juvenile polyp are not at increased risk of developing colorectal cancer and do not require further follow-up or investigations.[14,15]

SOLITARY PEUTZ–JEGHERS-TYPE POLYP

Solitary polyps, with the morphology that is characteristic of the hamartomas that arise in Peutz–Jeghers syndrome, are rarely seen in the colon.

Synonyms

None described.

Prevalence

These are excessively rare, only a few case reports have been documented in the literature.[16] Some of these cases may represent a particularly polypoid and arborizing form of polypoid mucosal prolapse (see p. 107 (Polypoid mucosal prolapse), below).

Endoscopic appearance and microscopic features

- These are identical to those seen in Peutz–Jeghers syndrome (see p. 135 in Chapter 6).

- Multiplicity of these lesions should, of course, raise the suspicion of the polyposis syndrome with its attendant gastrointestinal and extra-gastrointestinal neoplastic implications.

Biological behaviour and associated conditions

Solitary Peutz–Jeghers-type polyps are entirely benign and have no known neoplastic implication.

INFLAMMATORY POLYPS

Inflammatory polyps can be loosely defined as any polypoid structure developing consequent to inflammatory pathology.

They are a characteristic accompaniment of chronic ulcerative colitis but are also seen in Crohn's disease, diverticulosis and in some chronic infective conditions including schistosomiasis and amoebiasis.[17]

Iatrogenic, post-surgical polyps, whose pathogenesis can be considered to be post-inflammatory, are seen at anastomosis lines and at stomata. The pathology of these post-surgical polyps is usually simply that of an inflammatory polyp but occasionally there is a mucosal prolapse pathological component (see p. 106 (Polypoid mucosal prolapse), below).

The polyps that may occur at the site of a previous ureterosigmoidostomy may show features of inflammatory polyp (or indeed those of juvenile polyp) but the more clinically significant ureterosigmoidostomy polyps are adenomatous in type.[18]

Polyps with the features that are typical of inflammatory polyps may also be seen after previous ischaemic colitis and after radiotherapy.

Synonyms

Pseudopolyp. The use of this title is, in our view, to be discouraged. The term literally means a lesion that looks like a structure that protrudes above an epithelial surface: this is tautologous and nonsensical. In most other polyp terminology, the type is largely titled according to its pathogenesis and hence the use of the term 'inflammatory polyp' is advised.

Giant inflammatory polyp.

Prevalence

In strictly numerical terms, inflammatory polyps are probably the most prevalent of the large intestinal polyps. When cases of chronic inflammatory bowel disease are prone to the formation of such lesions, there are usually multiple inflammatory polyps, often numbering in excess of 100. There is little doubt that the more extensive the inflammatory bowel disease, especially ulcerative colitis, the more likely it is that inflammatory polyps will occur. Thus they are most often a reflection of the extent of the disease and the severity and number of acute relapses.

Clearly inflammatory polyps are only likely if there has been previous ulceration and subsequent regenerative change allowing the disorganised mucosa to become heaped up and polypoid.

Endoscopic and gross appearance

- The endoscopic appearance of inflammatory polyps is highly variable, depending on the cause of the lesions, their longevity and the presence of associated active inflammation.

- In active ulcerative colitis, the associated inflammatory change in relatively flat mucosa may be predominant with only small sessile elevations (Fig 5.5).

- In more chronic disease, subject to repeated relapses, more prominent polypoid structures develop (Fig 5.6).

- These polyps can be highly variable in shape and size. It is perhaps this variability which is the most characteristic feature of these polyps and helps to distinguish them from other polyps, in particular adenomas.

- Inflammatory polyps complicating both ulcerative colitis and Crohn's disease may be sessile or pedunculated. Because their pathogenesis relates to disordered regeneration of the mucosa after previous ulceration, they can take on remarkable appearances with the formation of mucosal bridges or become strikingly elongated or filiform with the appearance, almost, of multiple worms or spaghetti within the colon (Fig 5.6). These remarkable polypoid structures are most commonly seen in chronic ulcerative colitis. More commonly established inflammatory polyps appear finger-like with a bulbous tip. The latter can, on occasion, show ulceration and a cap of granulation tissue (Fig 5.7).

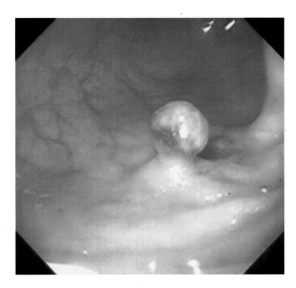

Figure 5.5 – Endoscopic appearance of an inflammatory polyp. It is pedunculated with a smooth surface.

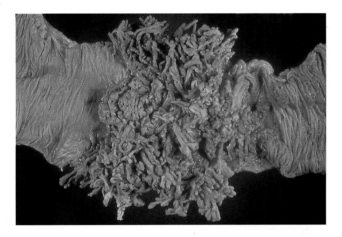

Figure 5.6 – The transverse colon in a patient with chronic ulcerative colitis. There are innumerable filiform polyps in a strictly localised segment of the colon.

Microscopic features

The commonest inflammatory polyps, those complicating ulcerative colitis and Crohn's disease, develop because the undermined mucosa at the edge of an ulcer regenerates excessively. The microscopic appearance is highly variable and depends on the time period since the acute attack of disease and the ulceration. Early inflammatory polyps feature plentiful granulation tissue, from the ulcer, and this may be excessive with a large cap of granulation tissue. More mature lesions are lined by intact, albeit architecturally distorted, mucosa (Fig 5.7).

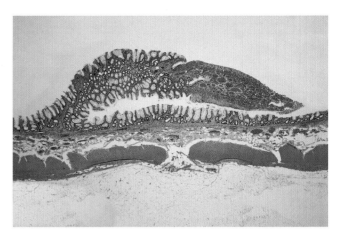

Figure 5.7 – A low power microphotograph showing filiform inflammatory polyp lined in part by mucosa and in part by granulation tissue (at right).

The mucosa of inflammatory polyps will show features of the disease that caused the polyp (Fig 5.8). For instance in ulcerative colitis there is gross crypt architectural distortion with dilatation and branching. In Crohn's disease, these architectural abnormalities are less marked but there may be other features of Crohn's disease, including granulomas.

Polyps occurring in diverticular disease are likely to show changes of mucosal prolapse. Indeed it seems likely that mucosal prolapse, and not inflammation *per se,* is the pri-

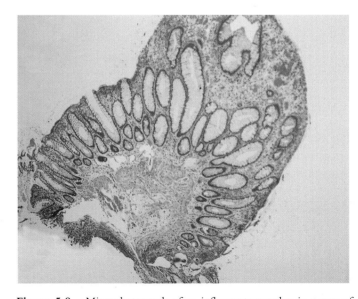

Figure 5.8 – Microphotograph of an inflammatory polyp in a case of chronic inflammatory bowel disease. There is increase in the depth and volume of the crypts and lamina propria. The latter may show fibrosis and an increase in the chronic inflammatory cell infiltrate.

mary pathogenic mechanism causing the development of polyps complicating diverticulosis.[19]

Inflammatory polyps occurring on a basis of radiation and ischaemia will demonstrate features of these diseases with vascular change being prominent in the former and dense fibrosis and mucosal distortion being prominent in both.

Post-infectious inflammatory polyps show variable features: those after previous bacterial infectious colitis show changes similar to those seen after ulcerative colitis.

In chronic intestinal schistosomiasis, the ova, either live or effete, of schistosoma may be readily demonstrated.

Biological behaviour and associated conditions

Inflammatory polyps have little clinical consequence apart from mimicry of more clinically significant polyps and the possibility that they may represent polypoid dysplasia in inflammatory bowel disease. Nevertheless multiple large inflammatory polyps, best called giant inflammatory polyposis, can occur, particularly in chronic ulcerative colitis but also occasionally complicating Crohn's disease, diverticulosis and schistosomiasis. Giant inflammatory polyposis can lead to bowel obstruction, excessive mucin secretion with electrolyte disturbances and even protein-losing colopathy.[20,21] The condition occasionally warrants segmental resection of the colon because of these complications.

METAPLASTIC POLYPS

Synonyms

Hyperplastic polyps, hyperplasiogenic polyps, inverted hyperplastic polyps.

Prevalence

Metaplastic polyps are the commonest polyps of the sigmoid colon and rectum, especially in the elderly, and they are usually multiple and are often clustered around rectal cancers.[22,23]

They are more common in males[24] and their frequency increases with age.[25,26]

They certainly account for the greatest number of patients who have large intestinal polyps and are the commonest polyp of the sigmoid colon and rectum. Some would maintain that, in strict numerical terms, inflammatory polyps are the more numerous.

They are found with the greatest frequency in patient groups with a high predilection for colorectal adenomas and adenocarcinomas and have a similar geographical and anatomical distribution to both adenomas and carcinomas.[27]

They share many histochemical features of adenomas and carcinomas. This has led some to speculate on their neoplastic potential.

Recent molecular evidence has suggested that, whilst they do show some molecular abnormalities in common with carcinoma, they also show differences and this has led to the current belief that these polyps represent a different histogenetic pathway and probably have little or no neoplastic potential.[25]

They remain one of the great enigmas of large intestinal pathology and have been a constant source of controversy particularly with regard to their neoplastic implication.

Endoscopic and gross appearance

- Metaplastic polyps appear endoscopically as pale nodules of the colorectal mucosa (Fig 5.9). They are most commonly small, usually less than 0.5 cm in diameter and sessile.

- They are characteristically, but not universally, situated on the apices of the mucosal folds of the colorectum.

- They usually appear to be rounded and irregular but occasionally are larger and more multilobate in shape. Size is not an absolute indicator of the nature of a polyp. Giant metaplastic polyps are well described and these may be in excess of 2 cm in diameter.[28]

Microscopic features

Metaplastic polyps show a similar configuration to normal colonic mucosa although the crypts within the polyps

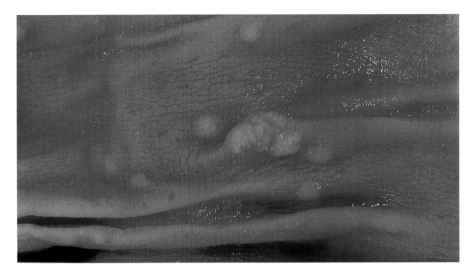

Figure 5.9 – A view of a colectomy specimen showing a cluster of typical pale metaplastic polyps.

appear longer than their normal mucosal counterpart and there is modest crypt dilatation. The most characteristic feature of metaplastic polyps, histologically, is their serrated surface (Figs 5.10 & 5.11).

They appear to represent a hypermaturation of the crypt epithelium, apparently due to a slowing of migration up the crypt, possibly associated with a delay in apoptosis at the epithelial surface.[23] This results in the distinctive excessive colonocytic and goblet cell accumulation, forming intraluminal papillary buds, and the serrated outline.

Unlike serrated adenoma (*vide infra*), metaplastic polyps show a relatively normal differentiation with the proliferative compartment (which often appears more prominent than in the adjacent normal colorectal mucosa) orientated basally and there being a well-defined basal–luminal gradient of differentiation.

In their classical form metaplastic polyps show no evidence of dysplastic change and thus have been regarded as hyperplastic or metaplastic phenomena rather than neoplasms.

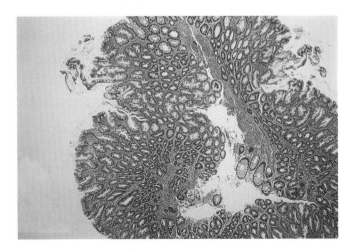

Figure 5.10 – This is a low power microphotograph of a metaplastic polyp. Note the irregular and villiform surface epithelium.

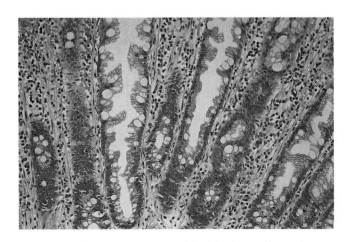

Figure 5.11 – This is a higher power view of the epithelial contour in a hyperplastic polyp.

Larger polyps can show more disquieting features. They can show villous change although not necessarily associated with dysplasia. Nevertheless these larger metaplastic polyps can harbour dysplastic foci with appearances that are identical to those of standard (usually tubular) adenomas. Combined adenomatous and hyperplastic (metaplastic) change is a distinctive feature of giant hyperplastic polyps.[28]

The combination of adenomatous and hyperplastic changes may be seen in adjacent areas, possibly representing adenomatous change in a pre-existing hyperplastic polyp or even a collision lesion. Alternatively the entire polyp can show features of both adenoma and metaplastic polyp and are then known as serrated adenoma (vide infra). For management purposes, both types of lesion should be regarded as adenomatous polyps.

Metaplastic polyps can show epithelial misplacement, especially those that are larger than 5 mm and when in the sigmoid colon. There remains a distinctive form of metaplastic polyp with florid epithelial misplacement. These are known as inverted hyperplastic polyps. They often show a right-sided colonic preponderance, a predominance in female patients, histological mimicry of both adenomas and carcinomas of the colon and multiplicity.[29,30] They often, macroscopically, show a puckered and pitted surface (presumably the result of underlying epithelial misplacement), surface mucus hypersecretion and underlying mucous cysts. In these inverted hyperplastic polyps, the epithelial misplacement is often seen closely related to lympho-glandular complexes, structures that are associated with an anatomical defect in the muscularis mucosae.[31] The most feasible mechanism for the development of inverted hyperplastic polyps would seem to be mild traction forces, due to the presence of the lesions on the apices of the mucosal folds, leading epithelial misplacement through these pre-existing defects in the muscularis mucosae.[30]

Biological behaviour and associated conditions

The close association, in anatomical, geographical and histochemical terms, of metaplastic polyp with adenoma and carcinoma has already been alluded to.

The size of metastatic polyps, even when multiple, is such that it is unwise to attribute any symptoms to these lesions.

Metaplastic polyps can be regarded as a marker, of relatively low specificity and sensitivity, for neoplastic change in the colon and rectum.

It has been suggested that metaplastic polyps in the distal colon and rectum are a 'sentinel' for adenomatous and carcinomatous change in the more proximal colon.[32] This has to be balanced against the fact that they are extremely common, especially in the elderly, and are thus of limited usefulness as such a marker.

The controversy concerning the metaplastic polyp's neoplastic potential has been vigorously debated. With the new molecular technology available, we now have some evidence that should be able to still this debate. Molecular abnormalities, akin to those seen in adenomas, have been described in metaplastic polyps: these include clonal chromosomal deletions, DNA microsatellite instability and K-ras mutations.[25,33,34] In one study about half of the metaplastic polyps showed K-ras deletions, a similar proportion to that seen in adenomas, but there was no evidence of mutations in the APC or p53 genes, which are characteristic molecular features of adenomas.[34] These findings strengthen the belief that metaplastic polyps may be benign neoplasms rather than hyperplastic overgrowths.[25] Unlike adenomas, however, metaplastic polyps do not usually harbour the critical molecular lesions that predispose to malignant progression (especially APC and p53 mutations). Similar molecular and morphological features are seen in aberrant crypt foci, microscopic colorectal crypt lesions that are also more commonly seen in colons with cancer. There is evidence to indicate that these lesions may progress to adenomas, if they have APC mutations, whereas the great majority regress by apoptosis.[33,35] It would seem likely that metaplastic polyps represent the macroscopic equivalent of such lesions with no significant malignant potential, per se, unless the polyp is above 1 cm in diameter or is associated with demonstrable adenomatous change.[25]

In conclusion we believe that metaplastic (hyperplastic) polyps should be regarded as a phenotypical expression of a different pathogenetic and molecular pathway compared to those of adenomas and carcinomas, with some similar histochemical and molecular alterations, in response to similar environmental stimuli. However they lack the molecular pathology that strongly predisposes to colorectal neoplasia. This would explain the pathological and epidemiological associations of metaplastic polyps with adenomas and carcinomas and, whilst noting the rare exceptions already identified, their apparently low malignant potential.

POLYPOID MUCOSAL PROLAPSE

The pathological concept of mucosal prolapse is now well accepted and the characteristic histomorphological features of fibromuscular proliferation within the lamina propria, epithelial hyperplasia, inflammation and ulceration are seen in a wide variety of clinical circumstances.[36] Firstly, the solitary ulcer syndrome, most commonly seen in the anterior aspect of the lower rectum in patients with defaecatory problems and pelvic floor descent, may cause polypoid mucosa and is, despite its name, neither always associated with mucosal ulceration nor are they always solitary.[37] Mucosal prolapse closer to the anal canal, often in association with haemorrhoids or other lesions of the anal canal, and particularly relating to gross and chronic disorders of defaecation and constipation, may lead to florid polypoid projection of the mucosa and this has been termed inflammatory cloacogenic polyp.[38] It is likely that so-called inflammatory myoglandular polyps,[39] which most commonly occur in the sigmoid colon, represent a manifestation of polypoid mucosal prolapse.[40,41]

Elsewhere in the colon, polyps due to mucosal prolapse can be seen in association with diverticular disease. In this situation, there is gross mucosal redundancy and the exaggerated propulsive forces, characteristic of diverticular disease, cause the mucosa to be propelled down the bowel to form polyps.[42] Mucosal prolapse mechanisms may be at play in the generation of polyps at ileostomies and colostomies although it should be emphasised that these polyps may be neoplastic, especially in familial adenomatous polyposis and in other conditions with a higher prevalence of neoplastic change.[43] Although strictly not within the large intestine, polypoid mucosal prolapse is also well described within the pelvic ileal reservoir, further underlining the potential relationship between mucosal prolapse and previous surgery.[44]

Synonyms

Prolapsing folds (diverticular disease), solitary ulcer (mucosal prolapse) syndrome, colitis cystica profunda, proctitis cystica profunda, inflammatory cloacogenic polyp, inflammatory myoglandular polyp.

Prevalence

This spectrum of diseases, all associated with the characteristic pathological features, are highly variable in prevalence. For instance, a degree of mucosal prolapse is inevitable in most cases of diverticular disease, and thus is extremely common in the elderly population. Classical solitary ulcer (mucosal prolapse) syndrome is distinctly rare and inflammatory cloacogenic polyp is also unusual, although both should be recognised by clinician and pathologist, not least because of their potential to mimic neoplasia.

Endoscopic appearance

- These conditions are so highly variable in their presentation and appearance that a general treatise on their endoscopic features is not appropriate. The classical presentation of solitary ulcer (mucosal prolapse) syndrome is with a single, rather flat ulcer on the anterior aspect of the rectum 5 cm above the dentate line. As already indicated, this is by no means universal and multiple ulcers, polypoid mucosa and extensive circumferential ulceration (although exaggerated on the anterior surface) may all be a manifestation of this syndrome.

- Inflammatory cloacogenic polyp has the greatest potential, both endoscopically and histologically, to be confused with other polyps, especially villous adenomas. It often appears, to the proctoscopist, as an ebullient, villiform, tumour mass at the anorectal junction.

Microscopic features

It would appear that fibromuscular proliferation within the lamina propria is one of the primary pathogenetic mechanisms because this is the most characteristic histological feature of all the diseases considered in this section (Fig 5.12). Inflammation, ulceration, granulation tissue caps, entrapment/misplacement of epithelium and proctocolitis cystica profunda are all seen but are variable and probably represent secondary effects (Fig 5.13).

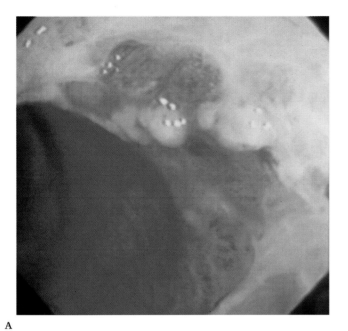

A

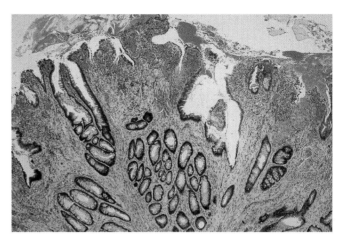

Figure 5.13 – At this power, the presence of crypt architecture disturbance and tear drop crypts with fibrosis and congestion is apparent. Note also the presence of necrotic slough 'capping' the lesion. It is the entrapment of glands within proliferative fibromuscular connective tissue, well seen here, that has potential for misinterpretation as malignancy.

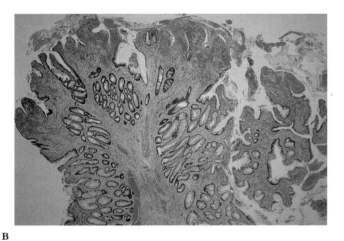

B

Figure 5.12 – (*a*) This shows the endoscopic appearance of solitary ulcer syndrome. Note the polypoidal configuration of the lesion in this case. (*b*) Low power magnification of a case of mucosal prolapse syndrome showing polypoid expansion, fibromuscular proliferation in the lamina propria and superficial ulceration.

Of all the polypoidal mucosal syndromes, inflammatory cloacogenic polyp is most liable to be mistaken for neoplasia, particularly tubulovillous adenoma, because of the florid villiform epithelial hyperplasia that is so characteristic.[45]

Solitary ulcer (mucosal prolapse) syndrome also has some potential for mimicry of neoplasia, because of the architectural distortion and epithelial misplacement that characterises the histology of the condition (Fig 5.13).

Biological behaviour and associated conditions

The variability of the clinical status of these conditions precludes a definitive statement on their behaviour. Suffice it to say that none have any major neoplastic potential. They need to be recognised to avoid erroneous diagnoses of neoplasia and for treatment of the underlying condition (most usually constipation and/or defaecatory anomalies).

ADENOMATOUS POLYPS

The adenoma is a benign neoplasm of colorectal epithelium and it is now well established that the adenoma–carcinoma sequence is the most important pathway for the genesis of colorectal cancer. Thus, adenomas are the most important of the large intestinal polyps because of their malignant potential. It should be emphasised, however, that whilst most carcinomas arise in a pre-existing adenoma, most adenomas (probably in excess of 95%) will not become malignant.

By definition adenomas are dysplastic: dysplasia has been defined as 'an unequivocal neoplastic alteration of the colorectal epithelium'.[46]

Adenomatous polyps are classified according to their histological morphology. The traditional classification divides adenomas into three subtypes: tubular, villous and tubulovillous. The former is the commonest and is characterised by a tubular morphology similar to that of the normal colorectal mucosa. However, the villous adenoma features finger-like processes, or villi, lined by neoplastic epithelium with a thin core of lamina propria. Most larger tubular adenomas have a degree of villous change and are referred to as tubulovillous adenomas. This classification is conventional but of limited use in clinical practice. Large-scale adenoma follow-up studies have demonstrated that the most important predictive factors for the development of malignancy within an individual polyp, and elsewhere in the colorectum, are its size, the grade of dysplasia and the amount of villosity (villousness).[47] Thus it would be more logical not to type adenomas, but to assess the amount of villosity to give a more accurate predictive analysis.

Although almost non-polypoid, and therefore not wholly within the scope of this text, some comment is appropriate on flat or depressed adenomas. There is increasing interest in these lesions for several reasons. Initially described from Japan,[48] these lesions were thought to be rare in Western endoscopic practice, accounting for less than 2% of adenomas and usually diagnosed only at the time of intestinal resection. Recent studies in the West have demonstrated that, using a stringent endoscopic technique, flat adenomas are considerably more common, accounting, in one unselected colonoscopic series, for 40% of all adenomas detected[49] and are more prevalent in younger patients in comparison to other adenomatous polyp types.[50] Flat adenomas exhibit higher grades of dysplasia than their protuberant equivalents, size for size, and also are much more likely to harbour foci of invasive malignancy. It has been suggested that these lesions have a different pathogenic and molecular evolution than standard adenomas and this may in part account for their apparently higher malignant potential.[51,52]

For the assessment of levels of invasion in such adenomatous polyps harbouring malignancy, the so-called Haggitt levels may be used; see p. 163.

Synonyms

Papillary adenomas, adenomatous polyps. These are the terminologies that were formerly applied to the tubular adenoma.

Prevalence

The prevalence of adenomas varies considerably, depending on the mode of assessment used, the geographical location, the age range of the patient group surveyed and the method of detection. For instance, colonoscopic surveys of average risk younger patients will give a prevalence rate of around 2% whilst necropsy studies, inevitably biased toward older populations, have shown rates of around 35% for males and 30% for females.[53]

As already indicated, colonoscopic surveys using dye-spraying techniques will detect considerably higher rates of flat adenomas than conventional techniques. Surveys have shown an increasing ratio of right-sided adenomatous (and carcinomatous) disease with time[54,55] and there are also differences in the left to right colonic disease ratio according to race.[56]

Endoscopic appearance

- The endoscopic appearances of adenomas are dependent upon the size, the type and, to some extent, the position of the polyp (Figs 5.14 & 5.15).

- Small adenomas (less than 3 mm) may be very difficult to see at endoscopy if they are in an awkward position or the visibility is in any way obscured. Small polyps tend to have the same appearance and colour as the adjacent mucosa or they may appear to be almost transparent.[56]

- Adenomas of intermediate size (between 5 and 10 mm) tend to appear redder than the adjacent mucosa and the colour and their surface appearances are helpful discriminators (Figs 5.14 and 5.15).

- Tubular and tubulovillous adenomas have a characteristic cerebral or sulcal appearance to their surface (particularly if the view is magnified) (Fig 5.16).[56]

- By the time an adenoma has reached a size of greater than 8 mm, the diagnosis becomes much more obvious endoscopically because adenomas, unlike metaplastic polyps, have a rich vascularity and they appear red and lobulated. At this size, tubular adenomas are usually stalked.

- In certain parts of the colon, especially the sigmoid, stalked polyps can become subject to propulsive forces resulting in torsion, ischaemia and ulceration. Thus ulceration and inflammation in a prominently stalked polyp is not necessarily an indicator of malignant change.

- Villous adenomas are more often sessile lesions (Fig 5.17). They can vary in size from small fronded and pale appearing excrescences, less than 5 mm in extent, to large carpeting lesions measuring in excess of 10 cm in diameter. The latter are most commonly seen in the rectum and, curiously, in the caecum, but are distinctly unusual in other parts of the colon.

- Smaller adenomas and flat adenomas are often difficult to visualize at the time of endoscopy. Dye-spraying techniques are of help here. Vital staining, using methylene blue or indigo carmine, helps to accentuate these adenomatous lesions.

- Adenomatous polyps, of all types, are also particularly accentuated when melanosis coli is present in the mucosa of the colon and rectum. The pigment of melanosis does not stain adenomatous polyps and thus they stand out as pale lesions against the brown/black mucosa.

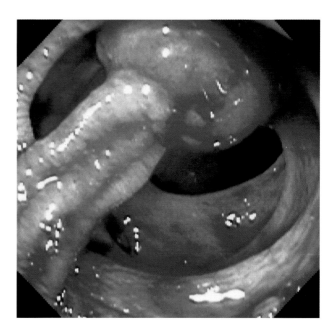

Figure 5.15 – A strikingly pedunculated adenomatous polyp, typically found in the sigmoid colon.

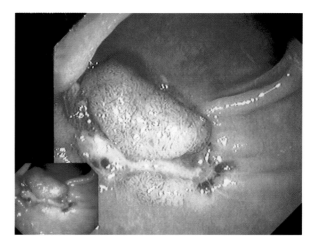

Figure 5.16 – A tubulovillous adenoma at endoscopy (both low power and with magnification). The sulcal appearance is seen on the surface.

Microscopic features

The polyp type determines the low power microscopic features of adenomas. Tubular adenomas consist of tightly packed tubules with variable amounts of lamina propria, the latter often considerably reduced compared with normal mucosa. The tubules may show branching, budding and dilatation, the latter particularly when a pedunculated polyp has been subject to mechanical forces. On the other hand

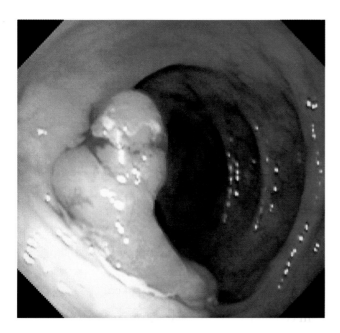

Figure 5.14 – The typical lobulated appearance of an average-sized adenoma in the transverse colon.

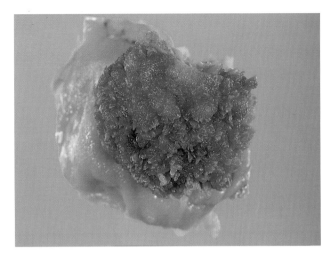

Figure 5.17 – A local excision specimen showing a sessile villous adenoma of the rectum.

villous adenomas show an exophytic morphology in which the dysplastic epithelium is thrown into folds (rather than villi, the term 'villous' here strictly being a misnomer) lined by dysplastic epithelium and containing a central core of lamina propria (Fig 5.18). Tubulovillous adenomas show features of both of these adenoma types (Fig 5.19).

All adenomas are dysplastic. They therefore show a disordered epithelial cell growth pattern with a failure of maturation and differentiation usually extending from the basal zone of the crypt to the surface of the lesion (Figs 5.19, 5.20 & 5.21).

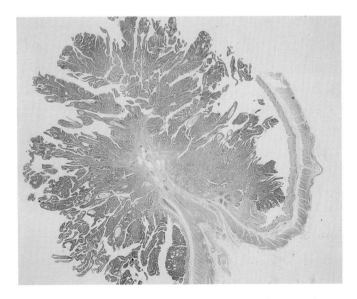

Figure 5.18 – A whole mount specimen of a case of villous adenoma showing the typical papillary cofiguration of the lesion.

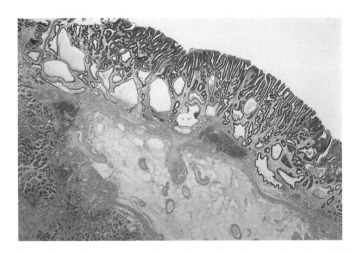

Figure 5.19 – Low power view of a tubular adenoma featuring mild dysplasia.

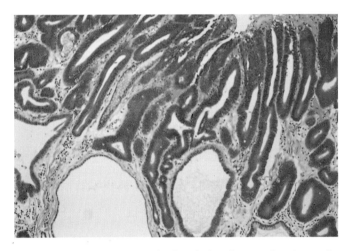

Figure 5.20 – Photomicrograph of a tubular adenoma showing moderate dysplasia.

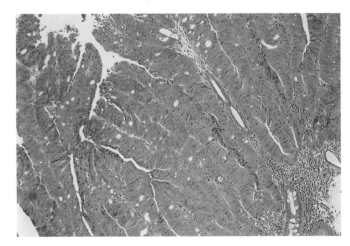

Figure 5.21 – A tubulovillous adenoma showing severe dysplasia contrasting with a single non-neoplastic crypt at bottom right.

Dysplasia within adenomatous polyps is still classified, for the most part, according to the method described by Konishi and Morson[57] into mild, moderate and severe dysplasia. This system has withstood the ravages of time and still provides a useful clinical and prognostic implication. Most small tubular adenomas show mild dysplasia with the entire tubule being lined by epithelium that is morphologically similar to that seen in the normal basal proliferative zone (Fig 5.19). The nuclei are enlarged, oval and hyperchromatic but orientation of nuclei remains toward the basement membrane. In moderate dysplasia the nuclear features are only a little more advanced but polarity is less well preserved with characteristic stratification of nuclei (Fig 5.20). In severe dysplasia, polarity is lost altogether and cytological changes are much more pronounced, the nuclei being enlarged and spheroidal with an open chromatin pattern and prominent nucleoli. In severe dysplasia there are architectural abnormalities with complex branching of dysplastic tubules and cribriform change (Fig 2.21). In other organs, such advanced cytological and architectural abnormality would warrant a diagnosis of carcinoma-in-situ or even intramucosal carcinoma. In many countries such a diagnosis is used (as in the 'TNM' classification; pathological stage pTis) but such a tumour does not appear to have any metastatic potential, one factor here being the relative paucity of intramucosal lymphatics in the colorectum.[58] In the UK, it is recommended that terms such as carcinoma-in-situ and intramucosal carcinoma are not applied to large intestinal pathology as they may precipitate unnecessary radical surgery.[59]

Misplacement or pseudoinvasion of adenomatous epithelium within the submucosa is a close mimic of invasive adenocarcinoma in pedunculated adenomas, especially those in the sigmoid colon which are more likely to undergo torsion, ischaemia and architectural distortion.[60] Useful pathological discriminators for a diagnosis of epithelial misplacement include the retention of lamina propria around dysplastic glands, a lack of morphological features of malignancy in the epithelium and signs to indicate mucosal ischaemia and haemorrhage, especially haemosiderin deposition.

Biological behaviour and associated conditions

Adenomas are usually entirely asymptomatic. Bleeding, sufficient to cause anaemia, is most unusual and will only occur in the larger polyps, particularly those in excess of 2 cm in diameter. Large villous adenomas can cause excessive mucus discharge per rectum and the very large carpeting villous adenomas can cause water and electrolyte disturbances.

Adenomas are important because of their malignant potential and their malignant implication. Thus, all polyps that could represent adenomas should be removed and submitted for histological assessment. The latter will give an indication of size, type and grade of dysplasia, all three of which are the most important predictive factors for the development of malignancy within that individual polyp and elsewhere in the colorectum.[47] The latter is particularly important: studies have demonstrated that adenomas within the rectum and sigmoid colon, and therefore readily detectable by flexible sigmoidoscopy, are important markers for adenomatous, and malignant, disease in the proximal colon.[61] Thus it is now believed that flexible sigmoidoscopy is an appropriate screening methodology for the detection of colorectal neoplasia, not only because distal adenomas can be sought and removed, but also because they themselves represent a marker for proximal colonic adenomatous disease, especially if the rectal and sigmoid adenomas are larger and of villous type.

The pathogenic and molecular factors that underpin the progression of adenomas to malignancy are largely beyond the scope of this text. Nevertheless this is an area of increasing importance, not only in basic science research, but also increasingly in clinical practice. The interested reader is referred to other texts for reference.[63–65]

Occasionally adenomatous polyps removed at the time of endoscopy may harbour foci of invasive adenocarcinoma: such a circumstance is fraught with management conundra, the decision to submit the patient to surgical resection often being especially vexatious. This subject is dealt with on p. 115 (Carcinomatous polyp (*vide infra*)), below.

SERRATED ADENOMA

The term serrated adenoma is given to a distinct form of polyp with histological features of both metaplastic (hyperplastic) polyp and adenoma. Thus there is clear histological evidence of dysplasia but there are also the characteristic features of metaplastic polyp. There remains some confusion about what exactly constitutes such a polyp not least because the term has been used reversibly with that of mixed adenomatous and hyperplastic polyp. This latter term should be reserved for polyps that show a juxtaposition of adenomatous and metaplastic (hyperplastic) features, not an uncommon feature in some of the larger adenomatous polyps. The term serrated adenoma should be reserved for those polyps in which there is evidence of both adenomatous and metaplastic (hyperplastic) change in each and every part of the polyp (Fig 5.22).

Synonyms

Mixed hyperplastic and adenomatous polyp (but see above for definitions).

Prevalence

When strictly defined as above, serrated adenoma is rare and probably accounts for less than 1% of all adenomatous polyps. They show a similar age distribution, being commoner in the elderly.[66]

Endoscopic appearance

- In general serrated adenomas show no obvious macroscopic differences to their much commoner standard adenomatous counterparts.

- They are usually single but on occasion can be multiple (up to seven have been described in a single patient).[66] They are of variable size, as might be expected, with some reaching more than 2 cm in size: these polyps are slightly more prevalent in the right colon.

Microscopic features

Histology shows features of both adenomatous and metaplastic (hyperplastic) polyps (Fig 5.22). Thus the polyps, which usually show a predominance of a tubular morphology, have a serrated outline, as seen in the metaplastic polyp, but also disclose goblet cell immaturity, upper zone

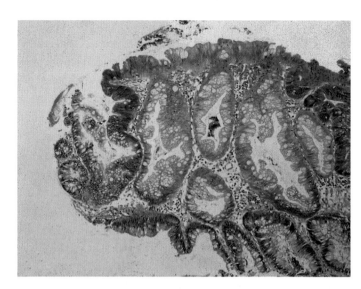

Figure 5.22 – A serrated adenoma showing clear evidence of variable adenomatous change but with a diffuse serration typical of metaplastic polyp.

proliferative activity and mitoses, and a lack of cytological maturity toward the epithelial surface.[66,67]

Biological behaviour and associated conditions

There have been few studies of the malignant potential of serrated adenomas. There have been two analyses of the proliferative activity within serrated adenomas and these have demonstrated the marked hyperproliferation throughout the crypts, akin to that seen in adenomas.[67,68] This, and circumstantial evidence from our study of cases, lead us to believe that, notwithstanding the highly characteristic histopathological features, these lesions should be considered as standard adenomas of the colon and rectum, with regard to dysplasia grading and overall management.

CARCINOMATOUS POLYPS

Carcinomatous polyps are defined as adenomatous polyps in which cancer has invaded, by direct continuity, through the muscularis mucosae and into the submucosa.[69] Invasive adenocarcinoma can be seen in two forms in polyps of the large intestine. Firstly, adenomatous polyps, removed at endoscopy, will occasionally harbour a focus of invasive adenocarcinoma, often in the centre of the polyp and extending into the stalk. Secondly, the entire polyp may be composed of adenocarcinomatous tissue with no obvious adenomatous component demonstrated. It is generally assumed that the latter lesion did once have an adenomatous component and that this has been destroyed by the carcinoma.

Synonyms

Malignant polyps.

Prevalence

The prevalence of adenocarcinoma arising in an adenomatous polyp is determined by three major factors, the size of the polyp, the amount of villosity and the grade of dysplasia. Thus, large carpeting villous adenomas are much more likely to harbour foci of invasive malignancy than small mildly dysplastic tubular adenomas. It should be remembered that small adenomas are relatively common whereas larger adenomatous polyps are rare. Thus just under 5% of all adenomas, in standard pathological practice, will show evidence of invasive malignancy.[70]

Polypoid adenocarcinomas are also rare in pathological practice. They account for less than 1% of invasive adenocarcinomas. They are usually very well delimited, without evidence of vascular spread and can often be effectively treated by local excision.

In one of the large series, it has been shown that none of the polyps that were 5 mm or less in size contained malignant components.[71]

Endoscopic and gross appearance

- Focal adenocarcinoma, in an adenomatous polyp, is most likely to be seen in polyps in the rectum and sigmoid colon. Whilst the phenomenon is more likely to occur in larger polyps, there may be few characteristic macroscopic features (Fig 5.23).

- Ulceration is certainly more common in malignant polyps but this may be seen in adenomas that are subjected to torsion forces, for example in the sigmoid colon, and does not necessarily imply that the polyp is malignant.

- Carcinomatous polyps are more likely to be irregular, to show bleeding from surface ulceration and to be firmer to endoscopic palpation and biopsy.[56] These signs of possible malignancy should alert the endoscopist to perform a thorough electrocoagulation of the base of the stalk, to ensure histopathological assessment of the stalk (and therefore the margin of excision) and to mark the site of the polyp with a tattoo, should histological evaluation result in a recommendation for surgical resection.[56]

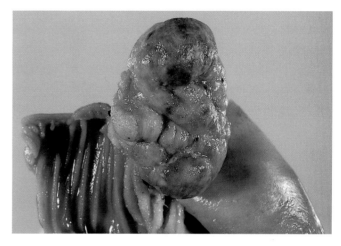

Figure 5.23 – A carcinomatous polyp showing solidity and ulceration at its tip, endoscopic features suspicious for malignancy.

Microscopic features

The diagnosis of adenocarcinoma demands the presence of architectural and cytological abnormalities within the epithelial component with clear and unequivocal evidence of invasion and an appropriate stromal reaction. Since resection may be the consequence of a diagnosis of malignancy, diligence on the part of the pathologist is important.

The diagnosis of malignancy requires evidence of invasion across the muscularis mucosae into the submucosa by neoplastic glands and/or cells (Fig 5.24). This should be accompanied by a stromal reaction in the form of tumour-associated fibrosis or desmoplasia.

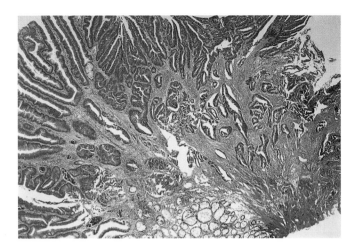

Figure 5.24 – A carcinomatous polyp. At top left is the adenomatous component whilst centrally there are invasive glands with a prominent desmoplastic reaction.

The cytological features of malignant epithelium are usually different to those of adenomas and thus the stromal and cytological features enable the pathologist to readily differentiate normally sited or misplaced adenomatous epithelium from invasive malignancy.

Pathological mimics of adenocarcinoma on biopsy are well recognised and include epithelial misplacement and colitis cystica profunda, the mucosal prolapse (solitary ulcer) syndrome and endometriosis.

Biological behaviour and associated conditions

The management of carcinomatous polyps, after initial endoscopic resection, remains controversial. The literature indicates that surgical conservatism is appropriate if the adenocarcinoma is not poorly differentiated, does not show involvement of vascular spaces and is well clear of the line of endoscopic diathermy excision (indicated by an eosinophilic coagulative necrosis zone).[72,73] In one study even the presence of vascular invasion did not appear to justify subsequent resection.[74] This is somewhat corroborated by the fact that, in resection specimens, submucosal vascular spread has no prognostic influence.[75] Nevertheless at least one large study has shown high rates of vascular involvement (17.6%) and that such a feature predicts likely local lymph node involvement.[73] It should be noted that *local* recurrence of adenocarcinoma after endoscopic polypectomy is not a major clinical problem: of greater importance is the possibility of local lymph node involve-

ment. We are well aware of cases in which the criteria for conservatism have been met, yet surgical resection has been undertaken and lymph node metastases have been demonstrated. As such Astler–Coller C1 cases have such a good prognosis (in comparison to Dukes C cases as a whole) and given the literature's equivocation, it is recommended that each case is judged on its own merits, particularly if the patient is relatively young and fit, in which case limited resection, to include the local lymphatic field, may well be justified. The controversies of various treatment modalities have been summarised in a recent review.[76]

POLYPOID CARCINOID TUMOURS

Carcinoid tumours are occasionally seen in the large intestine. They are the most common form of neoplasm in the appendix but they do not present as polyps and will not therefore be further considered. The proximal colon is a mid-gut structure and carcinoids arising here show macroscopic and microscopic features that are similar to those of carcinoids arising in the small intestine (see p. 81 in Chapter 4). Carcinoids arising in the left colon and rectum show the typical features of hindgut carcinoid with a characteristic histological appearance. They are almost always asymptomatic and are discovered during investigation for other anorectal conditions such as haemorrhoids, fissures and rectal carcinomas. It should be emphasised that carcinoid tumours may present as large ulcerating tumours and are not necessarily polypoid. Nevertheless rectal carcinoid, the commonest large intestinal neuro-endocrine tumour, is, in its commonest form, small and polypoid.

Synonyms

Neuroendocrine tumour. Entero-endocrine tumour.

Prevalence

Colonic carcinoid tumours are rare and most cases are described either in case reports or in small series. About 50% occur in the caecal area whilst the remaining parts of the colon account for a prevalence of about 10%.[77]

Rectal carcinoids are appreciably commoner than their colonic equivalents. Nevertheless they are still said to account for only 0.05% of all rectal tumours in one series.[78]

Small submucosal lesions may not be included in this series for these lesions are overwhelmingly the commonest manifestation of carcinoid tumour in the large intestine. Indeed some have suggested that rectal carcinoid may well be the commonest carcinoid tumour in the gut and it is only because these lesions are small and asymptomatic that they do not come to the attention of medical personnel.[79]

They appear to be appreciably commoner in males.[79]

Endoscopic appearance

- Caecal and colonic carcinoid tumours tend to be large lesions. They are in excess of 5 cm, on average, when malignant and still measure a mean of 4.7 cm when showing no evidence of metastatic disease.

- Ulceration is a very characteristic feature, whether exhibiting features of malignancy or not and this appears to be related simply to the size of these lesions.

- There are no absolutely characteristic macroscopic features that allow colonic carcinoids to be differentiated from colonic carcinomas.

- As already indicated, most rectal carcinoids are much smaller. They are generally round polyps with a size less than 13 mm in diameter, covered by a normal-appearing mucosa.[80] Often a faint yellow colour is visible endoscopically.[80] They may occur in the rectum of patients with ulcerative colitis and are then presumably a consequence of endocrine cell hyperplasia.[81] The larger, more often malignant, rectal carcinoid tumours show no features that allow them to be distinguished, macroscopically, from adenocarcinomas of the rectum.

Microscopic features

Carcinoid tumours arising in the caecum and right colon show morphological features similar to small intestinal lesions (see p. 82 in Chapter 4) (Figs 5.25 & 5.26). Thus, histologically, caecal and colonic carcinoids show the classical or insular pattern (A1 pattern of Jones and Dawson).[82]

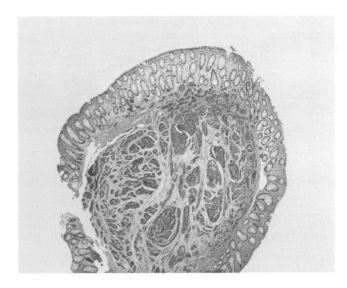

Figure 5.25 – A low power magnification of a polypoidal carcinoid tumour of the colon. Note the intact surface epithelium and the proliferation of the neoplastic cells beyond the muscularis mucosae.

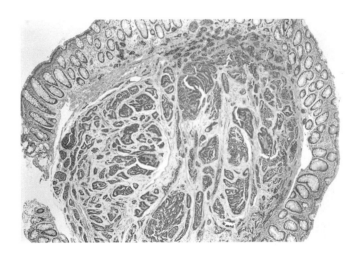

Figure 5.26 – High power magnification of the carcinoid tumour. Note the monotonicity of the neoplastic cells and the lack of pleomorphism.

Tubular differentiation may be seen and the tumours are usually both argyrophil and argentaffin. As with small bowel lesions, they are often extensively infiltrative within the wall of the intestine, commonly involving all four layers of the bowel wall. Vascular involvement is often a prominent feature.

The histology is very different for rectal carcinoids. These small lesions are usually the palisading, ribboning types of carcinoid (type B)[82] characteristic of the hindgut. Mixed types of carcinoid or tumours showing a predominant 'classical' pattern do occur. Nests of carcinoid tumour often infiltrate the mucosa and this is not a feature indicative of a more aggressive behaviour. The small rectal lesions never show ulceration. Rectal carcinoid tumours seldom show argentaffinity although they may show some argyrophilia. Although the great majority of rectal endocrine tumours are benign, it may be difficult on morphological grounds to distinguish these from more aggressive tumours.

Features that correlate with increased metastatic potential include size of the tumour (greater than 2 cm in diameter), ulceration, spread in the muscularis propria, extensive necrosis and an infiltrating growth pattern.[80,83,84] Cytological features that suggest malignancy include an anaplastic sheet-like morphology, nuclear pleomorphism and a high mitotic activity.[80,83,84] Nevertheless, many metastasizing rectal carcinoids show no cytological features that suggest malignancy, having the characteristic ribboning pattern with minimal cytological atypia. In these tumours the size, the presence of ulceration and the growth pattern may indicate increased aggressiveness.[83]

Other variants of endocrine tumours are extremely uncommon in the large intestine. Goblet cell carcinoid (adenocarcinoid) has been described in the colon, outside the appendix, but we have never seen an example.

Biological behaviour and associated conditions

Symptomatic colonic carcinoid tumours usually present with clinical features similar to those of colonic adenocarcinoma. Thus common presentations are with abdominal pain, change in bowel habit and the signs of large bowel obstruction.

Despite their mid-gut derivation and high rate of associated metastatic disease, carcinoid syndrome is much less common with colonic carcinoids, compared to small intestinal carcinoids. Carcinoid syndrome only occurs in about 5% of colonic carcinoid cases with extensive liver metastases. Rectal carcinoids, if large, will present with similar symptoms and signs to those of rectal carcinoma.

Management

As already indicated, most carcinoids are small submucosal polypoid nodules. These are not usually symptomatic and are usually discovered during rectal examination performed for other reasons. Such small rectal carcinoids are best treated by simple local excision.[80] More recently aspiration lumpectomy at the time of endoscopy has been advocated for these small rectal carcinoids.[85]

Larger lesions may demand more radical surgery as these have a high incidence of metastatic disease, although some have argued that the prognosis of such large, malignant tumours is poor regardless of the extent of surgery.[84]

BENIGN LYMPHOID POLYPS

Synonyms

Nodular lymphoid hyperplasia. Benign lymphoma (this is a poor term and should be avoided).

Prevalence

Nodular lymphoid hyperplasia is most commonly seen, in the gut, in the stomach, terminal ileum and rectum. It is best regarded as an exaggerated immune response to antigenic stimulus and usually affects many lymphoid aggregates resulting in the simulation of a polyposis syndrome (see p. 141 in Chapter 6). Isolated benign lymphoid polyps, representing a similar but localised exaggerated lymphoid response, are almost entirely confined to the rectum and such polyps elsewhere in the colon are exceptional.

Multiple small lymphoid polyps are a common accompaniment of inflammatory bowel disease (especially ulcerative colitis)[86] and diversion proctocolitis (Figs 5.27 and 5.28).[87]

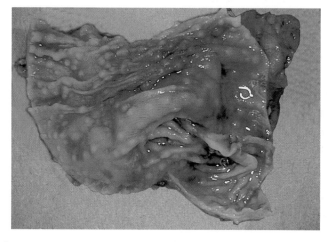

Figure 5.27 – A surgical specimen from a patient with faecal diversion showing large numbers of polypoid lesions in the rectum.

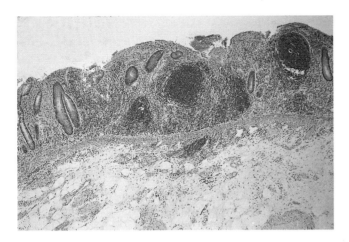

Figure 5.28 – A low power view of the rectum seen in Fig 5.27 showing the multiple lymphoid follicles that characterise the condition of diversion proctocolitis.

Sporadic/isolated lymphoid polyps are less common but are most often seen in children and young adults.

Endoscopic appearance

- Most benign lymphoid polyps occur in the more distal rectum and around the anorectal junction.[88] Here they probably represent an enhanced immune response to local infection/inflammation.

- They may be small sessile and multiple (Fig 5.27) but, more usually, they present as a single mass, measuring between 0.5 and 5 cm in diameter.

- They characteristically have a smooth and non-ulcerated surface.

Microscopic features

Histologically benign lymphoid polyps show an intact surface mucosa, either rectal or anal canal-type, although this may be compressed or attenuated by the submucosal mass (Fig 5.28).

The body of the polyp, within the submucosa, is composed of hyperplastic lymphoid tissue with multiple enlarged, geographic, lymphoid centres with prominent germinal centres.

On biopsy, differentiation from malignant lymphoma, especially that deriving from mucosa-associated lymphoid tissue ('MALToma') may be difficult. Helpful diagnostic features of a benign lymphoid polyp include its relatively small size, circumscription of the lesion, non-involvement of the muscularis propria, lack of ulceration and an absence of positive features of lymphoma, notably infiltration and destruction of epithelial structures ('lympho-epithelial lesions') and infiltration by cleaved lymphoid cells of germinal centres. If there is doubt, excision biopsy may allow a positive diagnosis to be made. Very occasionally molecular analysis is required to demonstrate the lack of immunoglobulin gene rearrangement, the characteristic molecular finding in B-cell lymphomas of the gut.

Biological behaviour and associated conditions

Benign lymphoid polyps of the rectum most commonly present with rectal bleeding despite the fact that the mucosa is usually intact over the polyp.

These lesions show no increased risk of malignant lymphoma.

Management

Excision is curative although many regress without resort to excision.

Any diagnostic doubt should encourage excision biopsy to fully refute the diagnosis of lymphoma.

OTHER LARGE INTESTINAL POLYPS

Although those polyps considered previously are the commoner polyp types liable to be encountered in routine endoscopic and pathological practice, there remain many other pathological entities that may present as a polypoid mass in the large intestine. These vary from benign connective tissue tumours, such as lipomas and gastrointestinal stromal tumours (GISTs: more often known as leiomyomas in the large intestine), through to malignant lesions such as metastatic malignant melanoma and Kaposi's sarcoma. Metastatic melanoma is a well-recognised mimic of polyposis syndromes, as it causes multiple relatively small submucosal masses that project into the bowel lumen. Kaposi's sarcoma, complicating AIDS, may involve the large intestine and presents as a bluish polypoid mass.

Malignant lymphoma may be polypoid, especially if low grade and localised. It is beyond the scope of this book to describe every lesion, whether neoplastic or not, that may present as a polypoid mass in the large intestine. Instead the following list provides an *aide-memoire* for those lesions which may, rarely, present to the endoscopist or pathologist as a polyp.

Non-neoplastic lesions. These include pneumatosis cystoides intestinalis (Figs 5.29 & 5.30), endometriosis, lipohyperplasia of the ileo-caecal valve, barium granuloma, oleogranuloma and malakoplakia.

Lymphoid/haematogenous neoplasms. These include malignant lymphoma and various leukaemias, especially myeloblastic sarcoma (tissue deposit of acute myeloblastic leukaemia).

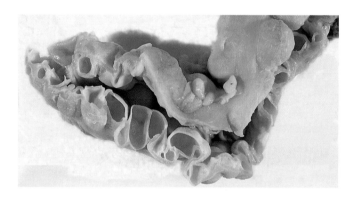

Figure 5.29 – A surgical specimen from a patient with pneumatosis coli. Note the relatively large submucosal cysts which often appear endoscopically as polyps.

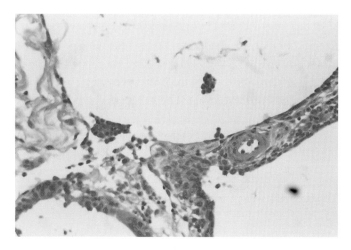

Figure 5.30 – The histology of pneumatosis coli in which the cysts are lined by histiocytes and some multinucleate giant cells.

Benign connective tissue tumours. These include neurofibroma, lipoma, neurilemmoma, inflammatory fibroid polyp, leiomyoma, gastrointestinal stromal tumour, ganglioneuroma and haemangioma.

Malignant connective tissue tumours. These include leiomyosarcoma, malignant gastrointestinal stromal tumour, liposarcoma, neurofibrosarcoma, angiosarcoma and Kaposi's sarcoma.

Metastatic tumours. These include malignant melanoma, metastatic lobular carcinoma of breast, other metastatic carcinomas, lymphoma and sarcoma.

Large pedunculated colonic polyp composed of mucosa and submucosa. This kind of polyp has only been identified as a separate entity in Japan.[89] They are characterised by being elongated, drumstick-shaped and measuring up to 16 cm in length. They can be seen anywhere in the colon. Histologically, there is intact mucosa overlying oedematous loose and fibrotic submucosal connective tissue. We believe that they are simple post-inflammatory polyps and question the categorisation as a separate entity.

REFERENCES

1. Jacoby RF, Schlack S, Cole CE, *et al*: A juvenile polyposis tumor suppressor locus at 10q22 is deleted from non-epithelial cells in the lamina propria. *Gastroenterology* 1997; **112**: 1398–1403

2. Heiss KF, Schaffner D, Ricketts RR, Winn K: Malignant risk in juvenile polyposis coli: increasing documentation in the pediatric age group. *J Pediatr Surg* 1993; **28**: 1188–1193

3. Mestre JR: The changing pattern of juvenile polyps. *Am J Gastroenterol* 1986; **81**: 312–314

4. Ansell ID, Vellacott KD: Colonic polyps complicating ureterosigmoidostomy. *Histopathology* 1980; **4**: 429–438

5. Groisman GM, Benkov KJ, Adsay V, Dische MR: Osseous metaplasia in benign colorectal polyps. *Arch Path Lab Med* 1994; **118**: 64–65

6. Williams GT, Arthur JF, Bussey HJR, Morson BC: Metaplastic polyps and polyposis of the large intestine. *Histopathology* 1980; **4**: 155–170

7. Billingham R, Bowman H, MacKeisan J: Solitary adenomas in juvenile patients. *Dis Colon Rectum* 1980; **23**: 26–30

8. Friedman CJ, Fechner RE: A solitary juvenile polyp with hyperplastic and adenomatous glands. *Dig Dis Sci* 1982; **27**: 946–948

9. Dajani YF, Kamal MF: Colorectal juvenile polyps: an epidemiological and histopathological study of 144 cases in Jordanians. *Histopathology* 1984; **8**: 765–779

10. Giardiello FM, Hamilton SR, Kern SE, et al: Colorectal neoplasia in juvenile polyposis or juvenile polyps. Arch Dis Childhood 1991; **66:** 971–975

11. Dickey W, Alderdice J, McConnell B: Dysplastic change in the solitary juvenile polyp. Endoscopy 1996; **28:** 641

12. Liu TH, Chen M-C, Tseng H-C: Malignant change of juvenile polyp of colon. A case report. Chinese Med J 1978; **4:** 434–439. (In English)

13. Jones MA, Hebert JC, Trainer TD: Juvenile polyp with intramucosal carcinoma. Arch Pathol Lab Med 1987; **111:** 200–201

14. Nugent KP, Talbot IC, Hodgson SV, Phillips RK: Solitary juvenile polyps: not a marker for subsequent malignancy. Gastroenterology 1993; **105:** 698–700

15. Kapetanakis AM, Vini D, Plitsis G: Solitary juvenile polyps in children and colon cancer. Hepatogastroenterology 1996; **43:** 1530–1531

16. Nakayama H, Fujii M, Kimura A, Kajihara H: A solitary Peutz–Jeghers-type hamartomatous polyp of the rectum: report of a case and review of the literature. Jap J Clin Oncol 1996; **26:** 273–276

17. Shepherd NA: Polyps and polyposis syndromes of the intestines. In Current Diagnostic Pathology, Henry K (ed.). Edinburgh, Churchill Livingstone 1997: pp. 222–238

18. Ansell ID, Vellacott KD: Colonic polyps complicating ureterosigmoidostomy. Histopathology 1980; **4:** 429–438

19. Kelly JK: Polypoid prolapsing mucosal folds in diverticular disease. Am J Surg Pathol 1991; **15:** 871–878

20. Anderson R, Kaariainen IT, Hanauer SB: Protein-losing enteropathy and massive pulmonary embolism in a patient with giant inflammatory polyposis and quiescent ulcerative colitis. Am J Med 1996; **101:** 323–325

21. Koga H, Iida M, Aoyagi K, et al: Generalized giant inflammatory polyposis in a patient with ulcerative colitis presenting with protein-losing enteropathy. Am J Gastroenterol 1995; **90:** 829–831

22. Goldman H, Ming S, Hickok DF: Nature and significance of hyperplastic polyps of the human colon. Arch Pathol 1970; **89:** 349–354

23. Williams GT: Metaplastic polyposis. In Familial Adenomatous Polyposis and Other Polyposis Syndromes, Phillips RKS, Spigelman AD, Thomson JPS (eds). London, Edward Arnold 1994: pp. 174–187

24. Williams GT, Arthur JF, Bussey HJR, Morson BC: Metaplastic polyps and polyposis of the large intestine. Histopathology 1980; **4:** 155–170

25. Arthur JF: The structure and significance of metaplastic nodules in the rectal mucosa. J Clin Pathol 1968; 21: 735–743

26. Williams GT: Metaplastic (hyperplastic) polyps of the large bowel: benign neoplasms after all? Gut 1997; **40:** 691–692

27. Cappell MS, Forde KA: Spatial clustering of multiple hyperplastic, adenomatous and malignant colonic polyps in individual patients. Dis Colon Rectum 1989; **32:** 641–652

28. Summer HW, Wasserman NF, McClain CJ: Giant hyperplastic polyposis of the colon. Dig Dis Sci 1981; **26:** 85–89

29. Sobin LH: Inverted hyperplastic polyps of the colon. Am J Surg Pathol 1985; **9:** 265–272

30. Shepherd NA: Inverted hyperplastic polyposis of the colon. J Clin Pathol 1993; **46:** 56–60

31. O'Leary AD, Sweeney EC: Lympho-glandular complexes of the colon: structure and distribution. Histopathology 1986; **10:** 267–284

32. Foutch PG, DiSario JA, Pardy K, et al: The sentinel hyperplastic polyp: a marker for synchronous neoplasia in the proximal colon. Am J Gastroenterol 1991; **86:** 1482–1485

33. Jen J, Powell SM, Papadopoulos N, et al: Molecular determinants of dysplasia in colorectal lesions. Cancer Res 1994; **54:** 5523–5526

34. Otori K, Oda Y, Sugiyama K, et al: High frequency of K-ras mutations in human colorectal hyperplastic polyps. Gut 1997; **40:** 660–663

35. Shpitz B, Hay K, Medline A, et al: Natural history of aberrant crypt foci – a surgical approach. Dis Colon Rectum 1996; **39:** 763–767

36. du Boulay CEH, Fairbrother J, Isaacson PG: Mucosal prolapse syndrome: a unifying concept for solitary ulcer syndrome and allied conditions. J Clin Pathol 1983; **36:** 1264–1268

37. Madigan MR, Morson BC: Solitary ulcer of the rectum. Gut 1964; **19:** 871–881

38. Lobert PF, Appelman HD: Inflammatory cloacogenic polyps. Am J Surg Pathol 1981; **5:** 761–766

39. Nakamura S, Kino I, Akagi T: Inflammatory myoglandular polyps of the colon and rectum. Am J Surg Pathol 1992; **16:** 772–779

40. Chetty R, Bhathal PS, Slavin JL: Prolapse-induced inflammatory polyps of the colorectum and anal transitional zone. Histopathology 1993; **23:** 63–67

41. Griffiths AP, Hopkinson JM, Dixon MF: Inflammatory myoglandular polyp causing ileo-ileal intussusception. Histopathology 1993; **23:** 596–598

42. Kelly JK: Polypoid prolapsing mucosal folds in diverticular disease. Am J Surg Pathol 1991; **15:** 871–878

43. Attanoos R, Billings PJ, Hughes LE, Williams GT: Ileostomy polyps, adenomas, and adenocarcinomas. Gut 1995; **37:** 840–844

44. Blazeby JM, Durdey P, Warren BF: Polypoid mucosal prolapse in a pelvic ileal reservoir. Gut 1994; **35:** 1668–1669

45. Saul SH: Inflammatory cloacogenic polyp: relationship to solitary rectal ulcer syndrome/mucosal prolapse and other bowel disorders. Hum Pathol 1987; **18:** 1120–1125

46. Riddell RH, Goldman H, Ransohoff D, et al: Dysplasia in inflammatory bowel disease. Standardised classification with provisional clinical application. Hum Pathol 1983; **14:** 931–966

47. O'Brien MJ, Winawer SJ, Zauber AG, et al: The National Polyp Study. Patient and polyp characteristics associated with high grade dysplasia in colorectal adenomas. Gastroenterology 1990; **98:** 371–379

48. Muto T, Kamiya J, Sawada T, *et al*: Small 'flat adenoma' of the large bowel with special reference to its clinicopathological features. *Dis Colon Rectum* 1985; **28**: 847–851

49. Rembacken BJ, Fujii T, Cairns A, *et al*: Flat and depressed colonic neoplasms: a prospective study of 1000 colonoscopies in the UK. *Lancet* 2000; **355**: 1211–1214

50. Lanspa SJ, Rouse J, Smyrk T, *et al*: Epidemiologic characteristics of the flat adenoma of Muto. A prospective study. *Dis Colon Rectum* 1992; **35**: 543–546

51. Fujimori T, Satonaka K, Yamamura IY, *et al*: Non-involvement of ras mutations in flat colorectal adenomas and carcinomas. *Int J Cancer* 1994; **57**: 51–55

52. Kubota O, Kino I: Depressed adenomas of the colon in familial adenomatous polyposis. Histology, immunohistochemical detection of proliferating cell nuclear antigen (PCNA) and analysis of background mucosa. *Am J Surg Pathol* 1995; **19**: 318–327

53. Williams AR, Balasooriya BA, Day DW: Polyps and cancer of the large bowel: a necropsy study in Liverpool. *Gut* 1982; **23**: 835–842

54. Gerharz CD, Gabbert H, Krummel F: Age-dependent shift-to-the-right in the localization of colorectal adenomas. *Virchows Arch A Path Anat Histopath* 1987; **411**: 591–598

55. Offerhaus GJ, Giardiello FM, Tersmette KW, *et al*: Ethnic differences in the anatomical location of colorectal adenomatous polyps. *Int J Cancer* 1991; **49**: 641–644

56. Cotton PB, Williams CB: Colonoscopy and flexible sigmoidoscopy. In *Practical Gastrointestinal Endoscopy*. Oxford, Blackwell Science 1996: pp. 263–264

57. Konishi F, Morson BC: Pathology of colorectal adenomas: a colonoscopic survey. *J Clin Pathol* 1982; **35**: 830–841

58. Fenoglio CM, Kaye GI, Lane N: Distribution of human colonic lymphatics in normal, hyperplastic and adenomatous tissue. *Gastroenterology* 1973; **64**: 51–66

59. Morson BC, Dawson IMP, Day DW, *et al*: Benign epithelial tumours and polyps. In *Morson & Dawson's Gastrointestinal Pathology*, 3rd edn. Oxford, Blackwell Scientific 1990: pp. 567

60. Muto T, Bussey HJR, Morson BC: Pseudocarcinomatous invasion in adenomatous polyps of the colon and rectum. *J Clin Pathol* 1973; **26**: 25–31

61. Read TE, Read JD, Butterly LF: Importance of adenomas 5 mm or less in diameter that are detected by sigmoidoscopy. *N Engl J Med* 1997; **336**: 8–12

62. Atkin WS, Morson BC, Cuzick J: Long-term risk of colorectal cancer after excision of rectosigmoid adenomas. *N Engl J Med* 1992; **326**: 658–662

63. Fearon ER, Vogelstein B: A genetic model for colorectal tumorigenesis. *Cell* 1990; **61**: 759–767

64. Gryfe R, Swallow C, Bapat B, *et al*: Molecular biology of colorectal cancer. *Curr Problems Cancer* 1997; **21**: 233–300

65. Kinzler KW, Vogelstein B: Lessons from hereditary colorectal cancer. *Cell* 1996; **87**: 159–170

66. Longacre TA, Fenoglio-Preiser CM: Mixed hyperplastic adenomatous polyps/serrated adenomas. A distinct form of colorectal neoplasia. *Am J Surg Pathol* 1990; **14**: 524–537

67. Kang M, Mitomi H, Sada M, *et al*: Ki-67, p53, and Bcl-2 expression of serrated adenomas of the colon. *Am J Surg Pathol* 1997; **21**: 417–423

68. Fujishima N: Proliferative activity of mixed hyperplastic adenomatous polyp/serrated adenoma in the large intestine, measured by PCNA (proliferating cell nuclear antigen). *J Gastroenterol* 1996; **31**: 207–213

69. Cooper HS: Surgical pathology of endoscopically removed polyps of the colon and rectum. *Am J Surg Pathol* 1983; **7**: 613–623

70. Coverliza S, Risio M, Ferrari A, *et al*: Colorectal adenomas containing invasive carcinoma. Pathological assessment of lymph node metastasis. *Cancer* 1989; **64**: 1937–1947

71. Nusko G, Mansmann U, Altendorf-Hofmann A, *et al*: Risk of invasive carcinoma in colorectal adenoma assessed by size and site. *Int J Colorect Dis* 1997; **12**: 267–271

72. Morson BC, Whiteway JE, Jones EA, *et al*: Histopathology and prognosis of malignant colorectal polyps treated by endoscopic polypectomy. *Gut* 1984; **25**: 437–444

73. Muller S, Chesner IM, Egan MJ, *et al*: Significance of venous and lymphatic invasion in malignant polyps of the colon and rectum. *Gut* 1989; **30**: 1385–1391

74. Geraghty JM, Williams CB, Talbot IC: Malignant colorectal polyps: venous invasion and successful treatment by endoscopic polypectomy. *Gut* 1991; **32**: 774–778

75. Talbot IC, Ritchie S, Leighton MH, *et al*: The clinical significance of invasion of veins by rectal cancer. *Br J Surg* 1980; **67**: 439–442

76. Haboubi NY, Scott NA: Clinicopathological management of the patient with a malignant colorectal polyp. *J Colorect Dis* 2000; **1**: 2–7

77. Berardi RS: Carcinoid tumors of the colon (exclusive of the rectum): review of the literature. *Dis Colon Rectum* 1972; **15**: 383–391

78. Caldorola VT, Jackman RJ, Moertel CG, Dockerty MB: Carcinoid tumours of the rectum. *Am J Surg* 1964; **107**: 844–847

79. Jetmore AB, Ray JE, Gathright JB, *et al*: Rectal carcinoids: the most frequent carcinoid tumor. *Dis Colon Rectum* 1992; **35**: 717–725

80. Matsui K, Iwase T, Kitagawa M: Small, polypoid-appearing carcinoid tumors of the rectum: clinicopathologic study of 16 cases and effectiveness of endoscopic treatment. *Am J Gastroenterol* 1993; **88**: 1949–1953

81. Gledhill A, Hall PA, Cruse JP, Pollock DJ: Enteroendocrine cell hyperplasia, carcinoid tumours and adenocarcinoma in long-standing ulcerative colitis. *Histopathology* 1986; **10**: 501–508

82. Jones RA, Dawson IM: Morphology and staining patterns of endocrine cell tumours in the gut, pancreas and bronchus and their possible significance. *Histopathology* 1977; **1**: 137–150

83. Burke M, Shepherd N, Mann CV: Carcinoid tumours of the rectum and anus. *Br J Surg* 1987; **74:** 358–361

84. Koura AN, Giacco GG, Curley SA, *et al*: Carcinoid tumours of the rectum: effect of size, histopathology, and surgical treatment on metastasis free survival. *Cancer* 1997; **79:** 1294–1298

85. Imada-Shirakata Y, Sakai M, Kajiyama T, *et al*: Endoscopic resection of rectal carcinoid tumors using aspiration lumpectomy. *Endoscopy* 1997; **29:** 34–38

86. Flejou JF, Potet F, Bogomoletz WV, *et al*: Lymphoid follicular proctitis. A condition different from ulcerative proctitis? *Dig Dis Sci* 1988; **33:** 314–320

87. Yeong ML, Bethwaite PB, Prasad J, Isbister WH: Lymphoid follicular hyperplasia – a distinctive feature of diversion colitis. *Histopathology* 1991; **19:** 55–61

88. Lloyd J, Darzi A, Teare J, Goldin RD: A solitary benign lymphoid polyp of the rectum in a 51 year old woman. *J Clin Pathol* 1997; **50:** 1034–1035

89. Matake H, Matsui T, Yao T, *et al*: Long pedunculated colonic polyp composed of mucosa and submucosa. *Dis Colon Rectum* 1998; **41:** 1557–1561

Polyposis Syndromes

N A Shepherd

INTRODUCTION

The term polyposis refers to a syndrome in which multiple polyps are a conspicuous feature. The term has been abused and misinterpreted. This is mainly because sporadic polyps are often multiple. *The term polyposis should be restricted to recognisable and strictly defined syndromes in which the primary feature is the presence of multiple polyps.* Defining a polyposis syndrome, however, may not be easy. In the commoner polyposis syndromes, especially familial adenomatous polyposis and juvenile polyposis, the definition primarily associates with the number of polyps, in the appropriate clinical setting with or without molecular confirmation. Some other 'polyposes', for instance metaplastic polyposis, possess no precise definition. The situation is complicated by the existence of mixed polyposis syndromes. Some of the latter, although apparently very rare, are relatively well defined in clinical, pathological and genetic terms.

The intention of this chapter is to concentrate only on those polyposis syndromes that are relatively well defined. There are conditions in which multiple polyps are found and in which the term polyposis may be used to describe these conditions, which are not part of the remit of this chapter. Most notable in this category is inflammatory polyposis. This acquired condition is possibly the commonest form of 'polyposis' but is highly variable in its cause, clinical presentation and implications. Multiplicity of inflammatory polyps has been considered in a previous chapter (see pp. 99–101 in Chapter 5). Furthermore various submucosal lesions, and tumours deeper within the bowel wall and outwith, can be multiple and present as a polyposis. Various stromal lesions, e.g. lipomas, ganglioneuromas and neurofibromas, can occur in multiplicity resulting in the simulation of a polyposis syndrome. There are other, acquired, conditions such as pneumatosis cystoides intestinalis and polypoid mucosal prolapse (see p. 101 and p. 109 in Chapter 5) that can characteristically present, especially in endoscopy, as a polyposis. Finally, and rarely, metastatic carcinoma and, in particular metastatic malignant melanoma, can present as polyposis when multiple deposits have seeded into the gastric and/or intestinal submucosa.

To some, the interest in polyposis syndromes in the medical community seems to be overplayed. This should be countered by the fact that one, familial adenomatous polyposis, is the most important *in vivo* model for the molecular and clinico-pathological study of colorectal carcinogenesis. We are learning more about the molecular basis of several of the polyposis syndromes and this is becoming more and more relevant to the day-to-day management of patients afflicted by these, often sinister, diseases. The defined structure of each preceding chapter is not applicable to the polyposis syndromes as these inevitably cut across the boundaries set by anatomy and therefore a revised layout has been used. This comprises Definition and genetics, Synonyms and associations, Prevalence, Molecular pathology, Oesophageal manifestations, Gastric manifestations, Small intestinal manifestations, Large intestinal manifestations, Endoscopic and gross appearance, Microscopic features, Extra-alimentary manifestations, Malignancy risk and Management.

FAMILIAL ADENOMATOUS POLYPOSIS

Definition and genetics

Familial adenomatous polyposis (FAP) is the commonest, best known and most important of the inherited polyposis syndromes.[1] *It is defined clinically by the presence of more than 100 adenomatous polyps in the colorectum.*[2] It was formerly known as familial polyposis coli but the realisation that adenoma proneness occurs throughout the stomach and intestines led to the change of title. The now well recognised gene that is mutated in the syndrome is, confusingly, known as APC (adenomatous polyposis coli): the reason for this simply relates to historical precedence, the initials FAP having already been appropriated by familial amyloidotic polyneuropathy.

In pathogenetic terms, it is of major importance as a model for the adenoma–carcinoma sequence, since FAP patients inherit a constitutional mutation of the APC gene and most patients will have developed one or more colorectal cancers by the age of 50 unless prophylactic colectomy is undertaken.

FAP is inherited on an autosomal dominant basis. Thus a propositus case will pass on a 50% risk of the disease to all his/her children.

Synonyms and associations

Adenomatous polyposis coli (APC); (Familial) polyposis coli.

Several syndromes are associated with adenomatous polyposis and represent varying phenotypic expression of APC gene mutations. Perhaps the best known is Gardner's syndrome, which associates adenomatous polyposis with epidermal cysts and odontomas of the jawbones.[3] The general belief, now, is that the use of the term Gardner's syndrome is confusing and should be discouraged, notwithstanding the importance of Gardner's original observations, because there are so many differing expressions of the disease due to the genetic abnormalities present. Many of the extra-intestinal associations are further described below (*vide infra*).

The association between intestinal polyposis and tumours of the central nervous system has been called Turcot's syndrome.[4] Turcot and colleagues described two siblings in whom multiple colonic polyps were associated with astrocytoma and medulloblastoma. In the past the existence of this syndrome has been controversial because of its phenotypic and genetic diversity. This can now be partially explained by the demonstration of two distinctive molecular abnormalities in patients with multiple colorectal adenomas and brain tumours: mutation of the APC gene in cases with FAP phenotypic expression and a propensity to cerebellar astrocytoma and mutation of a mismatch-repair gene with a proneness to high grade astrocytoma.[5]

Prevalence

FAP is the foremost inherited polyposis syndrome, whose prevalence (at about 1 in 10 000) is remarkably consistent throughout the world.[6] It should be noted, however, that the phenotypic expression of the disease varies, according to both the site of mutation in the APC gene (which is thus similar within afflicted families) and according to environmental influences. Thus, in certain Eastern countries, where gastric adenomas and carcinomas are commoner because of environmental factors, notably *Helicobacter* prevalence and diet, the prevalence of such gastric lesions is also enhanced in FAP patients.

Molecular pathology

The APC gene was localised to chromosome 5q more than 10 years ago[7] and it has subsequently been identified and sequenced.[8] The cDNA predicts a protein of 2843 amino acid residues with no obvious signalling regions, transmembrane domains or nuclear targeting sequences, indicating its cytoplasmic localisation.[9] The product of the APC gene associates with the adherens junction proteins, alpha, beta and gamma catenins, and it has been suggested that this association mediates growth regulatory signals.[10,11] Thus, mutant APC may allow inappropriate transcriptional activation in colorectal tumours.[12,13]

Whilst an all-encompassing review of the molecular pathology of FAP is beyond the scope of this chapter, a short resumé of progress in the diagnostic and pathological relevance is appropriate. Commercial gene tests are now available for FAP.[14] In combination with ocular fundic examination for Congenital Hypertrophy of the Retinal Pigment Epithelium (CHRPE, which occurs in more than 80% of affected individuals), a confident diagnosis of the disease can be made without resorting to sigmoidoscopy, especially in younger children in whom polyps may not be detectable, yet, in the colorectum.[15] Nevertheless, whilst these techniques may well become the mainstay of diagnosis in the future, in most centres the diagnosis still depends upon sigmoidoscopic assessment and histological confirmation.

It is becoming increasingly apparent that the site of mutation in the APC gene may influence the phenotype of the disease.[16,17] This may have important implications for patient management. For instance, it has been shown that patients with mutations beyond codon 1250 have considerably less rectal failure (usually rectal carcinoma development) after previous ileorectal anastomosis (IRA) and it is suggested that mutation analysis may be used to determine the surgery performed (IRA versus total proctocolectomy and pelvic ileal reservoir).[18] The occurrence of both desmoid disease and CHRPE may also be determined by the APC gene mutation site[19] although it should be emphasised that the association between mutation site and phenotype is not absolute.[20]

Oesophageal manifestations

None well delineated.

Gastric manifestations

The commonest gastric manifestation of FAP, especially in Western countries, is the fundic gland cyst polyp.[21] These small fundic polyps are regularly seen outside the syndrome and represent a common form of polyp in the stomach. They are usually considered to be hamartomatous but very similar histological features may be seen in small hyperplastic/regenerative polyps in the fundus (see p. 35 in Chapter 2). In FAP they are usually seen in multiplicity. In the same Western populations, adenomas and carcinomas, in FAP patients, are unusual. In countries where these tumours are more prevalent, notably Japan and Korea, adenomas and carcinomas are a considerable problem in FAP.[22,23]

Small intestinal manifestations

Whilst duodenal adenomas have been recognised in FAP for more than a century, their significance has only been appreciated more recently.[24] The periampullary region of the duodenum is, after the large bowel, the commonest site for adenoma development in FAP. More than 90% of FAP patients will either have endoscopically demonstrable adenomas or will have histologically demonstrable microadenomas on random biopsies of the duodenal mucosa.[25] The St Mark's Hospital Polyposis Registry has developed a scoring system, now known as the Spigelman system, to classify the extent of duodenal adenomatous involvement based on the size, number, villosity and grade of dysplasia of the duodenal adenomas.[26] The Spigelman score has been shown to worsen significantly with time from diagnosis of FAP.[27] This underpins the importance of endoscopic assessment of the duodenum as the FAP patient gets older. Close surveillance is now recommended from the age of 25.[26]

The importance of duodenal pathology in FAP is emphasised by the fact that duodenal carcinoma has now become the commonest cause of death in FAP.[28] Controversies remain, nevertheless, about the optimal treatment for duodenal disease in FAP. Ablative techniques, including laser and photo-dynamic therapy, and pharmacological manipulation, especially with sulindac, have met with limited success whilst pancreaticoduodenectomy has to be considered to be over-treatment if duodenal carcinoma has not yet interceded. Endoscopic removal is often difficult, since the lesions are sessile and often carpeting, and has had little success in reducing the neoplastic risk.

Adenomatous polyps occur elsewhere in the small bowel. Relatively low numbers are seen in the terminal ileum,[29] although the occurrence of microadenomas have been recently described there.[30] Adenomas are also found in the pelvic ileal reservoir, after total colectomy and restorative proctocolectomy, but these do not appear to have much malignant potential despite the propensity of the ileal mucosa in the reservoir to undergo colonic phenotypic change.[31] Of more concern is the potential for neoplastic change of any remaining rectal mucosa adjacent to the ano-pouch junction, the cuff.[32]

Large intestinal manifestations

The macroscopic and histological features of large intestinal involvement in FAP are well known and are described in detail elsewhere.[33] FAP is effectively defined by the presence of more than 100 adenomatous polyps in the colon and rectum but, in practice, many more are usually present such that the mucosa is festooned with innumerable polyps, often numbering in excess of 2000. The disease is usually left side predominant and the diagnosis can be effectively established by flexible sigmoidoscopy and polyp biopsy. To make the diagnosis beyond any reasonable doubt, it is recommended that at least six rectal and sigmoid polyps are biopsied. Adenomatous polyps may not be apparent until late childhood or early adulthood[1] and apparent rectal sparing with a predominant right colonic disease can also occur.[34] In these circumstances, multiple random biopsies of the rectum and sigmoid colon, at the time of the initial sigmoidoscopy, and the demonstration of unicryptal and oligocryptal microadenomata may help to confirm the diagnosis of FAP.[34] In line with other phenotypic abnormalities in FAP, it would seem that the number and site of adenomas in the colon might correlate with the locus of the APC gene mutation.[20]

Whilst classical polypoid adenomas are the most usual manifestation of FAP, flat/depressed adenomas do also occur: it has been intimated that these are especially prevalent in one variant of the disease.[35] Flat adenomas have higher grades of dysplasia, relative to size, and probably a higher malignant potential. It is therefore especially important for endoscopists to be aware of these lesions. They need to be vigilant in their detection, using dye-spraying techniques for instance, when endoscopic surveillance is being undertaken, particularly in those patients who have had a colectomy and retain their rectum. The presence of flat adenomas is one of the factors that accounts for high rectal failure rates in FAP.[33]

The association of FAP with prevalent extra-intestinal manifestations, particularly CHRPE, and the delineation of the molecular pathology of the disease have made the establishment of the diagnosis, before the advent of endoscopically detectable polyps, relatively easy. Before this, and for pathogenetic reasons, scientists had sought to detect a phenotypic abnormality in the non-neoplastic colorectal mucosa of FAP patients. These studies had used methods as diverse as proliferative activity, mucin histochemistry, biochemical assays for the proliferation-associated enzyme ornithine decarboxylase and immunohistochemistry with monoclonal antibodies.[24] There does appear to be a proliferative abnormality of the non-adenomatous mucosa of FAP, which remains of some relevance in cell biological investigation.[36,37] Nevertheless there is little diagnostic advantage to be gained from these analyses because of the genetic advances in the diagnosis and management of FAP.

Endoscopic and gross appearance

- Despite the large numbers of polyps that characterise this disease, they are usually asymptomatic.

- The clinical diagnosis depends on endoscopic assessment and biopsy of representative numbers of the polyps. This cannot be over-emphasised as many syndromes and diseases can mimic FAP. Perhaps the best known mimic is lymphoid polyposis, an entirely benign condition, which occurs in children, and has been described in the otherwise unaffected offspring of FAP patients.[38]

- In established disease, the endoscopic appearances are characteristic.

- The rectal and colonic mucosa show multiple small polyps, usually less than 1 cm in diameter.

- There are occasional much larger polyps (Figs 6.1 & 6.2). The presence of ulceration in these larger polyps is a sinister feature and one that usually presages malignancy.

- Larger polyps and carcinomas (Fig 6.3)

are most likely to be seen in the rectum and left colon but right-sided predominance does occur.

- For full assessment, prior to a decision on the timing of colectomy, full colonoscopy is essential.

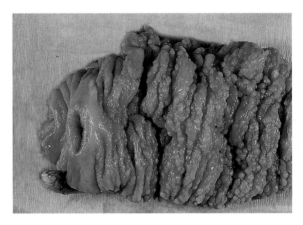

Figure 6.1 – A surgical specimen from a case of FAP. Note the mucosa is carpeted with numerous variously sized polyps.

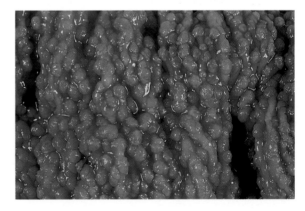

Figure 6.2 – A higher power view of the same case as that shown in Fig 6.1.

Microscopic features

The histopathology of adenomas, in all parts of the gut, has been described in detail on p. 41 in Chapter 2, and p. 108 in Chapter 5, and need not be further discussed. Microadenomas, however, are a histological feature that is

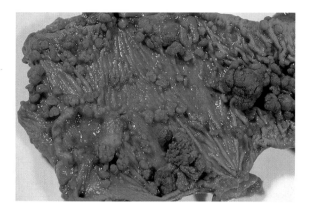

Figure 6.3 – A case of FAP in which an ulcerating carcinoma is associated with numerous large and small adenomatous polyps.

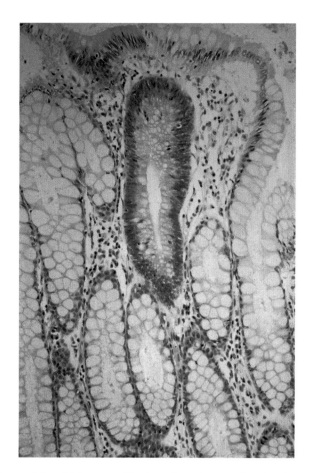

Figure 6.5 – Higher magnification of a unicrypt polyp showing mild dysplasia.

highly characteristic of, and diagnostically almost exclusive to, FAP (Fig 6.4). They are usually only seen in the large bowel mucosa or in the duodenum, although they have been recently described in the terminal ileum. They may be monocryptal, in which adenomatous change affects just one crypt, the adjacent crypts appearing histologically normal (Fig 6.5). As the lesion increases in size, due to crypt fission, the adenoma becomes firstly bicryptal and then oligocryptal. Only once it has reached a size when it is composed of about 10 crypts will it be demonstrable endoscopically and on examination of a resection specimen.

Extra–intestinal manifestations

Since affected individuals have a constitutional mutation or deletion of a gene that seems to be important for growth regulation, it is not surprising that FAP is associated with

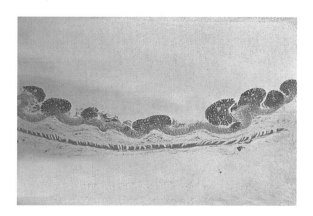

Figure 6.4 – A lower power magnification of the colonic section showing large numbers of small neoplastic polyps separated by normal mucosa.

disease outside the gastrointestinal tract. Some of these associations, such as that with minor soft tissue and bony lesions termed Gardner's syndrome, do not have a highly significant clinical implication. Others, especially desmoids and certain malignancies, do have profound clinical and prognostic implications for FAP patients. Conversely the FAP-associated retinal pathology, CHRPE, is important for its usefulness in FAP diagnosis rather than any clinical significance *per se*. Like other manifestations of FAP, it may be associated with specific locus mutations of the APC gene.[19] APC gene dysfunction appears to be particularly relevant to those tissues that are subject to the effects of bile and its metabolites, such as the duodenal and colorectal mucosa. Thus, adenomas and carcinoma have also been described in the extrahepatic bile ducts, the gall bladder and the pancreatic ducts in FAP patients.[39] In one series of routine cholecystectomies performed in FAP patients, foci of adenomatous dysplasia were disclosed in 40% of patients.[26]

Desmoid disease is probably the most significant and problematic of the extra-intestinal manifestations of FAP. Between 8 and 15% of patients with FAP have clinically significant fibromatoses or desmoids. Women are particularly affected, suggesting the possibility of hormonal influences. Familial clustering of FAP patients is also well described indicating that specific APC gene defects predispose to desmoid disease.[19] Fibromatoses may be found in musculo-aponeurotic sites in FAP patients but the clinically significant desmoids are those occurring either in the wall of the abdomen or within, principally in the retroperitoneum and mesentery. Presentation with intra-abdominal desmoid disease is particularly associated with surgery, the onset, often with rapid growth, frequently being 1 or 2 years after colectomy.[40] Desmoid disease is one of the leading causes of morbidity and mortality in FAP patients who have undergone prophylactic surgery.[41] In one series of FAP-associated intra-abdominal desmoids, the 5-year survival rate was only 68%.[40]

Desmoids are highly vascular and this feature accounts for the high frequency of life-threatening haemorrhage during surgery, a property that makes many experienced surgeons reluctant to attempt excisional surgery.[41] Medical treatment of desmoids has not been wholly successful: there have been mixed reports of the responses to steroids, anti-oestrogenic agents, non-steroidal anti-inflammatory agents (especially sulindac) and radiotherapy.[40] Trials of intensive chemotherapy are also underway.

Associations have been described between FAP and bone osteomas, epidermal cysts and other benign skin tumours, dental cysts and odontomas, thyroid tumours, hepatoblastoma, multiple endocrine adenomatosis (MEA) type IIb, pituitary adenomas, islet cell tumours, tumours of the adrenal cortex and various soft tissue tumours. The interested reader is referred to Brett et al[42] for a review of these associations. Pathologists will note the association between FAP and thyroid tumours.[43,44] Originally thought to be papillary in type, it is now clear that these tumours are a distinct type of follicular cell tumour. Features of papillary carcinoma, such as grooved nuclei and papillary architecture, are not consistent.[44] Furthermore, the tumours show appearances that are unusual for papillary carcinoma such as cribriform pattern and solid areas with a spindle cell component: the distinctive histological appearances should alert the pathologist to the possibility of associated FAP.[44] These tumours are well demarcated but often multifocal.[44]

Because of multicentricity, total thyroidectomy is advocated.[44] The carcinoma, unlike papillary carcinoma, is associated with metastatic disease or death in about 10% of cases.[44]

Management

If the colon of FAP patients is left *in situ*, then almost all patients will develop colorectal cancer by the age of 50. Therefore prophylactic colectomy remains the mainstay of FAP treatment. Whether the preferred operation is total colectomy and ileorectal anastomosis or restorative proctocolectomy and pelvic ileal reservoir is dependent on the age of the patient, patient preferences and the amount and controllability of rectal disease. As already indicated, genetic analysis may aid the surgical choice. If ileorectal anastomosis is the chosen alternative, then the patient requires rectal surveillance by regular sigmoidoscopy. Success in controlling rectal adenomas has been described with various pharmacological interventions, of which the most successful is probably the non-steroidal anti-inflammatory agent, sulindac.[45] This drug exerts its effects by the activation of apoptosis through prostaglandin inhibitory pathways.[46] The management of other manifestations of FAP has been discussed previously, above.

JUVENILE POLYPOSIS

Definition and genetics

Juvenile polyposis (JP) was first described in 1954 but was not really characterised until 1964.[47] The earlier literature is confusing as FAP and JP were frequently mistaken and even now there are well defined kindred that show features of both FAP and JP.[48] A practical definition of JP should include at least one of the following:[49,50]

- More than five juvenile polyps.

- Juvenile polyps throughout the gastrointestinal tract.

- Any number of juvenile polyps with a family history of JP.

Patients fulfilling these criteria fall into three main groups: (i) JP of infancy, (ii) JP throughout the gastrointestinal tract with or without a family history, (iii) JP of the colon (juvenile polyposis coli) (JPC) with or without a family history. The latter condition appears to be the commonest.[50] The syndrome of gastric juvenile polyposis has been recently proposed (see p. 28 in Chapter 2).

JP of infancy is extremely rare and has a very poor prognosis. Infants present with bleeding, diarrhoea, rectal prolapse, malnutrition, dehydration and large numbers of typical juvenile polyps in the colon. Death usually occurs at an early age.[51] Congenital defects, outside the colon, are more likely to occur in sporadic JP and about 20% of these patients will disclose congenital anomalies such as malrotation of the bowel, Meckel's diverticulum, mesenteric lymphangioma, congenital heart disease, hypertelorism and hydrocephalus.[52]

Infantile JP occurs on a sporadic basis and, given its association with multisystemic abnormalities, is presumably the result of major genetic deletion. Familial JP shares with FAP an autosomal dominant predisposition. Nevertheless a family history of the condition is only obtained in 20–50% of patients suggesting high rates of new mutations.[50]

Synonyms and associations

Several syndromes show polyps with superficial morphological similarities to those of juvenile polyps. Cronkhite–Canada syndrome polyps are similar but lack the pedunculated nature of colonic juvenile polyps: the conditions are easily differentiated by the presence of the ectodermal changes that are a *sine qua non* for the diagnosis of Cronkhite–Canada syndrome and the very different age distribution.

There are some overlaps between JP and Cowden's syndrome.[53] The latter describes the association between polyposis and cutaneous tumours with an increased propensity to tumours of the breast and thyroid. Current molecular evidence suggests that both conditions are associated with mutations of the long arm of chromosome 10 and hence overlap is not surprising. There are rare syndromes with similarities to both JP and Cowden's syndrome, which probably represent variants of these two conditions. The term Bannayan–Riley–Ruvalcaba syndrome has been proposed to reflect the clinical overlap between three such conditions, Bannayan–Zonana syndrome, Riley–Smith syndrome and Ruvalcaba–Myhre–Smith (RMS) syndrome.[54]

Prevalence

JP is considerably rarer than FAP and its true prevalence is difficult to define because of the uncertainties in the definition of the disease and because of overlap with other syndromes, most notably Cowden's syndrome. 1 in 100 000 is probably a reasonable estimate of its true prevalence.

Molecular pathology

To define the molecular abnormality in JP, initial attention was given to the APC gene but it has been shown that mutations of that gene were not responsible for familial JP.[55] Subsequently cytogenetic study of a case in which JP was associated with multiple congenital abnormalities has suggested that mutation of a tumour suppressor gene located on chromosome 10 (10q22.3q24.1) is the genetic abnormality in JP.[56] Further polymerase chain reaction (PCR) studies have demonstrated that this novel tumour suppressor gene is deleted/mutated in sporadic juvenile polyps and in JP.[57] Fluorescent *in situ* hybridisation (FISH) has demonstrated that the cells affected by the deletion/mutation reside exclusively in the lamina propria, and not in the epithelium, implying that the primary molecular abnormality, ostensibly, is in lamina propria cells. This would help to explain the characteristic morphological features of juvenile polyps.[58] Given these findings, it is of note that histological abnormality of the lamina propria of the non-polypoid mucosa of the colon has been recently described: in this series JPC was characterised by a fine nodular mucosa consisting of dense inflammation with slight crypt architectural abnormalities and a diffuse population of mixed inflammatory cell infiltrates in the superficial third of the lamina propria.[58] Whether these changes are specific or indeed sensitive for JPC requires further analysis of other patients with JPC.

Studies of the molecular changes that accompany dysplasia in the colonic polyps of JP have shown that dysplasia is associated with similar genetic defects, loss of p21, APC mutation, K-ras mutation and p53 overexpression, that are seen in sporadic forms of colonic neoplasia.[59]

Oesophageal manifestations

None that have been well defined.

Gastric manifestations

Gastric involvement in JP is second in importance only to colorectal involvement, in terms of symptomatology and malignancy risk. Anaemia and protein loss are common clinical accompaniments of gastric involvement.[60,61] The antrum is the commonest site of involvement although proximal extension of polyps is well recognised.[60,62] As with FAP, malignancy in gastric JP seems to be more common in those countries with a relatively high rate of sporadic gastric neoplasia, notably Japan.[60,61]

Small intestinal manifestations

Polyps do occur in the small intestine of JP patients. However clinical features and neoplastic risk are less significant here than in other parts of the alimentary tract.[50] There are reports of significant polyposis occurring in the pelvic ileal reservoir of JP patients.[63,64] In one of these cases,[63] three polyps were found to harbour dysplasia. Therefore the ileal pouch of JP patients should be regularly surveyed for polyp formation.[63]

Large intestinal manifestations

The large bowel is the most important organ of involvement by JP, particularly because of the malignancy risk (*vide infra*). Rectal bleeding is the most likely presentation although these subjects are often discovered by colonoscopic screening and are asymptomatic from their colorectal involvement. The polyps are multiple but number many less than those seen in FAP, usually between 50 and 200 (Fig 6.6). Different patients, and different families, show

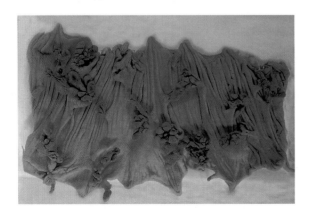

Figure 6.6 – Gross appearance of juvenile polyposis.

varying distributions of polyps. In the majority of JP cases, no particular segment is more likely to harbour polyps, the distribution being relatively even throughout the colon and rectum. In some kindred a distinct right-sided preponderance is seen.[64]

Endoscopic and gross appearance

- Colonoscopic examination shows distinctive changes because some, larger, polyps show very characteristic macroscopic appearances.

- Most polyps have the features of sporadic juvenile polyp (see p. 95 in Chapter 5), (Fig 6.6 and Fig 6.7) there are larger polyps, often measuring up to 5 cm in diameter, which possess a long stalk of normal-appearing mucosa and are composed of a number of smaller lobules all joined to the common stalk.

- This multilobulate, almost papillary, morphology is distinctive of the *atypical juvenile polyp* that characterises the syndrome.

Microscopic features

Most of the polyps resemble a typical sporadic juvenile polyp: however about 20% of polyps show different features.[65] These polyps, termed *atypical juvenile polyps*, have, despite their name, rather characteristic, morphological features which reflect their endoscopic and macroscopic appearances (Fig 6.7). They are multilobated, lack surface ulceration and show a papillary configuration. These polyps do not possess the abundant lamina propria that is so characteristic of classical juvenile polyps, although some resemble a lobulated cluster of closely packed juvenile polyps.[50]

Whereas dysplasia is exceedingly rare in sporadic juvenile polyps, the situation is very different in JP. Epithelial dysplasia occurs in three forms. Firstly, adenomatous polyps do occur in JP but these are unusual. Secondly, polyps show mixed features with the changes of both adenoma and juvenile polyp.[66,67] Thirdly, however, the most common presentation of dysplasia is within atypical juvenile polyps (Fig 6.8). Data from the St Mark's Hospital Polyposis Registry has shown that dysplasia is most common within these atypical juvenile polyps. In a review of 87 JP patients,

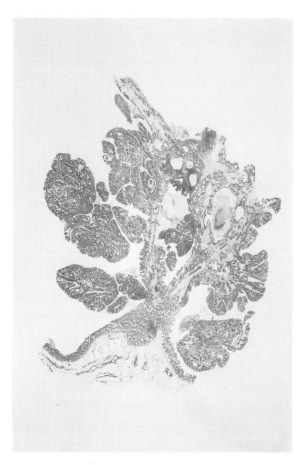

Figure 6.7 – Low power whole mount section of an atypical juvenile polyp. Note the papillary projections of the surface epithelium.

46% of atypical polyps showed dysplasia, 17% also displaying either moderate or severe dysplasia.[65] These data indicate that dysplasia and, therefore probably, carcinoma, does occur within the polyps of JP, and particularly within atypical juvenile polyps.[65]

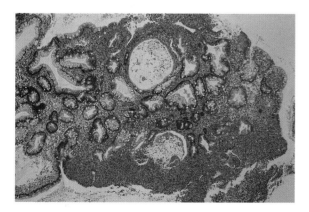

Figure 6.8 – An atypical juvenile polyp showing areas of dysplastic change.

Extra-alimentary manifestations

Extra-intestinal manifestations of JP are recognised but, unlike FAP, are poorly categorised.[68] They are most likely to be seen in infantile JP and in sporadic JP. About 20% of sporadic JP patients have congenital anomalies such as malrotation of the bowel, Meckel's diverticulum, mesenteric lymphangioma, congenital heart disease, hypertelorism and hydrocephalus.[52]

Malignancy risk

JP was originally thought to have little malignant potential.[47] It is now recognised that JP, and in particular JPC, has a very high risk of gastrointestinal, especially colorectal, malignancy. Earlier reports hinted at a concerning prevalence of gastrointestinal malignancy[69] but it was not until the report from the St Mark's Hospital Polyposis Registry that the true risk became apparent.[65] In this series of 87 JP patients, there was a colorectal cancer incidence of 14.6%. The median age of patients developing cancer was 32 years and many of these tumours were mucinous and poorly differentiated with an associated poor prognosis.[65] Genetic analysis of this data suggests a cumulative risk of cancer development, by the age of 60, of 68%.[70] Subsequent reports have served to confirm the high prevalence of malignancy in colorectal JP.[64,71,72]

Management

First and foremost, JP necessitates regular endoscopic screening, probably of both upper and lower tracts, for the patient and for asymptomatic first-degree relatives for diagnosis and because of the increased risk of malignancy, especially in the large bowel. Once the diagnosis is firmly established, the management of JP depends on the polyp load, particularly in the colon. Polyp removal is advocated, at all sites, because of the now clear documentation that dysplasia and, therefore, presumably, malignancy, does arise within the polyps themselves. In the stomach and colon, this can usually be achieved by gastroscopy and colonoscopy, respectively, although large polyps may require open, or perhaps, laparoscopic surgery, with gastrotomy/colotomy or even limited resection to remove them. In the small bowel, enteroscopy has been used to remove polyps.[73]

The role of prophylactic surgery, of the colon in particular, remains uncertain. This decision is largely dependent upon the controllability of the disease by endoscopic means and whether the patient or affected family members are particularly prone to neoplastic change in the polyps. If this is the case, then a case can be made for prophylactic colectomy. In one series subtotal colectomy was followed by rapid recurrence of the disease in the rectum and sigmoid colon, despite the disease having been mainly right-sided initially.[64] Restorative proctocolectomy would seem the best option in this situation as the small intestine appears to have a low neoplastic potential in JP. Disease recurrence in the pelvic ileal reservoir has been described in JP[63] and thus continued surveillance is undoubtedly required.

PEUTZ–JEGHERS SYNDROME

Definition and genetics

Unlike other polyposis syndromes, Peutz–Jeghers syndrome (PJS) is relatively easy to define because of the association of gastrointestinal polyposis with mucocutaneous pigmentation, especially in and around the mouth. Peutz[74] from Holland first described this relationship and Jeghers and his colleagues produced their timeless description of the syndrome in 1949.[75]

Like FAP and JP, PJS shows an autosomal dominant inheritance.

Synonyms and associations

Peutz syndrome, gastrointestinal polyposis with mucocutaneous pigmentation.

Prevalence

PJS is much rarer than both FAP and JP. Its estimated prevalence is 1 in 200 000.[76]

Molecular pathology

As in FAP and JP, there has been progress in the identification of the genetic basis of PJS. Initially possible target genes were thought to reside on chromosomes 1 or 6.[77] However, comparative genomic hybridisation of Peutz–Jeghers polyps, combined with loss of heterozygosity studies, has mapped a likely target gene to chromosome 19.[78]

Oesophageal manifestations

Polyps have also been described in the nasopharynx[74,79] and these may involve the upper oesophagus.

Gastric manifestations

Polyps do occur in the stomach but these are less common than in the small and large intestines. Rather perversely, gastric neoplasia is well described in Western populations[80,81] whilst in Japan, a country with a high prevalence of gastric malignancies, colorectal cancer appears to be the commonest malignant complication of PJS.[82,83] Solitary Peutz–Jeghers-type polyps are occasionally seen in the stomach in the absence of the syndromic features.[84]

Small intestinal manifestations

PJS polyps are most common in the small intestine. Peutz–Jeghers polyps of the small intestine commonly present with mechanical obstruction and can cause intussusception. Thus it is recommended that every attempt be made to remove larger polyps in the small bowel.[76] Nevertheless their removal may present considerable difficulties: enteroscopy is not particularly successful and often laparotomy or laparoscopic surgery and enterotomy is required to remove them.

The mechanical pressures induced by the presence of a large polyp within a viscus of a relatively small diameter can lead to obstructive pathology. Rarely duodenal polyps can cause biliary obstruction. In the small intestine, these mechanical pressures, as a result of obstruction and/or intussusception, probably account for the epithelial misplacement that is seen exclusively in small intestinal polyps.[85] This feature, also known as *enteritis cystica profunda*,[86] occurs in about 10% of small intestinal polyps and can closely mimic invasive malignancy.[85] Misplacement of the hyperplastic epithelium can be seen in the submucosa, muscularis propria and the subserosa. The latter is associated with cyst formation and puckering and induration, all features that suggest malignancy to the surgeon at the time of laparotomy or laparoscopic excision of small bowel polyps. Since there is also pathological mimicry of malignancy, it may well be that epithelial misplacement accounts for the exaggeration of the carcinomatous risk in PJS that characterises the earlier literature.[2]

Large intestinal manifestations

The large intestine is the second commonest site of involvement in PJS after the small bowel. The polyps share macroscopic and histological features to those seen elsewhere and can reach a considerable size: polyps up to 5 cm in size are not unusual. Obstruction of the large intestine is much less common than in the small bowel although intussusception of a small intestinal polyp may involve the proximal colon.

Endoscopic and gross appearance

- The polyp load, in stomach, small intestine and large intestine, is much less than in FAP although it is a highly variable feature.

- Some polyps can reach a considerable size (Fig 6.9) and complete endoscopic removal may not be possible.

- Given the low prevalence of dysplasia and malignancy within individual polyps, piecemeal removal, at endoscopy, may be justified.

Microscopic features

Although Peutz–Jeghers polyps are classified as hamartomas, they show a very organised architecture (Fig 6.10). They have a central core of smooth muscle that shows conspicuous branching, each branch being covered by mucosa of the type native to that part of the bowel in which the polyp arises. The mucosa of the polyp appears either morphologically normal or mildly hyperplastic. There is normal maturation of epithelial cells as they ascend the crypt toward the surface and, under normal circumstances, there is no evidence of dysplasia. Rarely solitary, sporadic polyps, identical to those seen in PJS, occur in the stomach, small intestine and large intestine.

Although there are occasional reports of dysplasia and frank carcinoma within classical Peutz–Jeghers polyps in PJS[82,87,88] dysplasia appears to be an uncommon phenomenon in classical Peutz–Jeghers polyps. In the St Mark's series, a review of 491 polyps showed no evidence of dysplasia in any of them.[85] Follow-up over 45 years of 48 PJS patients at the Mayo Clinic failed to reveal dysplastic change in any polyp.[89] There is one report from Japan documenting dysplasia and adenomatosis in 16% of polyps.[90] In view of the data from St Mark's and the Mayo Clinic, we would regard this as a spuriously high rate of neoplastic change that is not reflected in data from Western PJS series.

Extra-alimentary manifestations

Polyps have been described, outside the alimentary tract, in the nose and nasopharynx[74,79] and the ureter[91] but these are

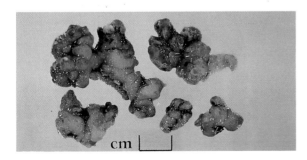

Figure 6.9 – Peutz–Jeghers syndrome. Macroscopic appearance of Peutz–Jeghers polyps from the small intestine, showing the characteristic lobulated appearance.

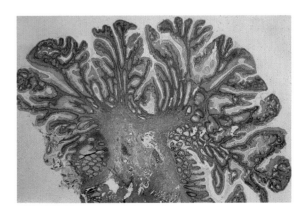

Figure 6.10 – Low power whole mount view of a Peutz–Jeghers polyp showing the branching of smooth muscle and the villiform appearance of the surface epithelium.

unusual and not of great clinical significance. Muco-cutaneous pigmentation, especially around the lips and in the mouth, is a pre-requisite for the diagnosis and the pathological basis for this is a melanin hyperpigmentation of the basal epidermal layer without an excess of melanocytes.

Of more importance is the wide range of tumours associated with PJS. Whilst some reports probably represent chance associations, there is little doubt that there is an increased risk of tumours of the breast, pancreas, ovary, testis and cervix in PJS. High prevalence rates of pancreatic and breast carcinomas, the latter often bilateral, are seen in PJS and it is recommended that PJS patients undergo surveillance for the early detection of cancers at these two sites.[76] Scully[91] first described the association between PJS and an unusual ovarian lesion, 'sex cord tumour with annular tubules' (SCTAT), a tumour thought to arise from granulosa cells but with a morphological pattern like that of Sertoli cells. The tumour may have oestrogenic effects, leading to endometrial hyperplasia. A well differentiated variant of endocervical adenocarcinoma, formerly known as *adenoma malignum*, is also closely associated with PJS and SCTAT.[92] Young and his colleagues have also described a functioning ovarian sex cord tumour that is apparently unique to PJS.[92] It is now thought likely that most female patients with PJS have small SCTAT tumours if the ovaries are diligently examined. They are usually small, bilateral and benign. Males with PJS are not immune from genital neoplasia: Sertoli cell tumours of the testis appear to represent a true complication of PJS. Whilst these are usually benign, they are associated with feminisation, especially presenting with gynaecomastia.[76]

Malignancy risk

Despite the low frequency of dysplastic change in the polyps of PJS, it is now clear that, like FAP and JP, there is an increased risk of gastrointestinal malignancy in PJS. The early literature is confusing and contradictory whilst sequential communications from the large PJS series at the Mayo Clinic have espoused a low cancer risk and surgical conservatism.[89,93] However, in a large Japanese series of 222 patients, there was a 13% incidence of gastrointestinal carcinoma.[83] More recently an 18-fold excess of cancer at all gastrointestinal sites has been described.[94] The St Mark's Hospital Polyposis Registry holds records of 72 PJS patients: nine have developed gastrointestinal malignancies, three in the stomach, four in the duodenum and jejunum and two in the colon.[88] The mean age at cancer diagnosis was 35.[88]

Management

It is clear that there is an increased risk of gastrointestinal malignancy in PJS and the majority of cancers, in the West at least, occur in the stomach and upper small bowel. Whilst surgical conservatism has been advocated in the past,[89] the excess risk of gastrointestinal malignancy would appear to demand a more aggressive approach to surveillance: it is now recommended that patients undergo biannual gastroscopy, colonoscopy and small bowel radiographical examination and that all polyps over 1.5 cm are removed. Gastric and colorectal polyps are usually removable at endoscopy whilst small bowel polyps may be excised at enteroscopy. Open or laparoscopic surgery may be required to remove the larger polyps of the small intestine.[76]

METAPLASTIC POLYPOSIS

Definition and genetics

Metaplastic polyposis (MP) is perhaps the most enigmatic and ambiguous of the polyposis syndromes. Metaplastic polyps themselves are usually multiple and thus there is a considerable dilemma in the definition of the polyposis. Indeed there have been few attempts to adequately define the syndrome, if such a syndrome does exist. Instead the literature merely describes cases in which multiple, mostly in excess of 50 in number, frequently large, metaplastic polyps occur in the large bowel, sometimes in association with focal adenomatous change and sometimes carcinoma, often in younger, frequently male, adults.[95–99] It should be emphasised that these MP cases are very rare and a diagnosis of MP *should not* be made in those elderly patients who have multiple small metaplastic polyps in association with adeno-carcinoma.

Synonyms and associations

Hyperplastic polyposis, giant hyperplastic polyposis, inverted hyperplastic polyposis.

Prevalence

Metaplastic polyposis, specifically that which occurs in young male adults and is possibly associated with colorectal cancer, is exceptionally rare. There are less than 20 cases in the entire world literature. There is a report of a single kindred with familial giant hyperplastic polyposis.[100]

Molecular pathology

Whilst progress has been made in our understanding of the molecular pathology of sporadic metaplastic polyps (see p. 106 in Chapter 5) MP is too poorly defined and too rare for any significant progress to have been made in the molecular changes that may predispose to this condition.

Oesophageal, gastric and small intestinal manifestations

None recognised.

Large intestinal manifestations

Most reports have indicated a diagnosis of MP when there have been more than 50 polyps present. In Williams' original report,[95] the maximum number of polyps was 156, although it is acknowledged that the number is likely to have been underestimated. Unlike sporadic metaplastic polyps, which are usually concentrated in the rectum and sigmoid colon, in MP the polyps show a more uniform distribution throughout the large intestine.[99] Most of the polyps are small, measuring less than 0.5 cm in diameter, although occasional polyps are larger than 1 cm.[95]

There are occasional reports of so-called giant hyperplastic polyposis.[100,101] A single kindred has been described in which giant hyperplastic polyps were associated with colorectal neoplasia, both adenomas and carcinomas. This seems to be a very rare familial syndrome associating giant hyperplastic polyps with high rates of colorectal cancer.

Inverted hyperplastic polyposis describes the presence of multiple large metaplastic-type polyps, exclusively in the right colon, which show epithelial misplacement and mucin hypersecretion.[102] They have a characteristic macroscopic appearance with a puckered and pitted surface (presumably the result of underlying epithelial misplacement), surface mucus hypersecretion and underlying mucous cysts. The epithelial misplacement is closely related to lympho-glandular complexes and it has been postulated that mild traction forces, due to the presence of the lesions on the apices of the mucosal folds, cause epithelial misplacement through these pre-existing defects in the muscularis mucosae.[102]

Endoscopic appearance

- Most of the polyps seen in MP are small and show the endoscopic features of sporadic metaplastic polyps.
- The larger polyps tend to be pedunculated.[95]

Microscopic features

The histological appearances of small polyps in MP do not significantly differ from sporadic metaplastic polyps. The larger polyps are more likely to be stalked, with a villous architecture and show epithelial misplacement,[95] a feature characteristic of inverted hyperplastic polyposis.[102] The several reports of MP also attest to the likely adenomatous change that may be an accompaniment of the metaplastic features.

Extra-alimentary manifestations

None recognised.

Malignancy risk

Given the young age of some of the MP patients with associated carcinoma, it is tempting to speculate that the presence of MP was directly responsible for cancer development. The complete disappearance of MP following treatment (resection and chemotherapy) of cancer in two patients suggests that the opposite is the case and possibly that the cancer is trophic to the polyps.[103]

The single kindred with familial giant hyperplastic polyposis has, it seems, a highly significant neoplastic risk, but it remains unclear whether this risk is directly related to the metaplastic/hyperplastic polyps.[100] The risk of malignancy in all patients with multiple metaplastic polyps probably relates not to the metaplastic polyps themselves but to the presence of adenomatous change in the polyps: this seems to occur especially in polyps over 1 cm in diameter.[104] It is important that all such lesions are subjected to histological assessment, not only to confirm or refute the presence of adenomatous change but also to rule out FAP, which is often the suggested clinical diagnosis.[104]

Management

It is not possible to make general recommendations about MP because the condition is so rare and unpredictable. The taking of an adequate family history is mandatory to rule out familial giant hyperplastic polyposis. Each case needs to be judged on its own merits, taking into account the age, sex, polyp load and whether any of the polyps demonstrate adenomatous change. Endoscopic surveillance is appropriate if all of these factors are favourable.

CRONKHITE–CANADA SYNDROME

Definition and genetics

The Cronkhite–Canada syndrome (CCS) is characterised by multiple polypoid excrescences of the gastrointestinal tract in association with characteristic skin and nail changes, namely alopecia, onycholysis and pigmentary changes.[105] It is an acquired, sporadic syndrome, which presents in late adulthood: gut involvement is often revealed by protein and electrolyte loss from the polyps.[106]

Synonyms and associations

The polyps of juvenile polyposis show superficial similarities to CCS although the polyps of CCS lack the pedunculated nature of colonic juvenile polyps. The two conditions are easily differentiated by the presence of the ectodermal changes of CCS and the very different age distribution.

Prevalence

CCS has a world-wide distribution and there is no familial tendency. The mean age at presentation is about 60 with a slight male preponderance. It is extremely rare and the average endoscopist or pathologist is only likely to see one case in their career.

Molecular pathology

Nothing is known of the molecular pathology of CCS but it has been intimated that the disease is due to the failure of normal epithelial cell proliferative mechanisms throughout ectodermal tissues resulting in hypoplasia of the skin and gut epithelium.[107]

Oesophageal manifestations

Approximately 2% of patients will show polypoid change in the oesophagus.[106]

Gastric manifestations

Almost all patients (96% in one series)[106] show gastric involvement. The lesions may resemble those of Menetrier's disease, both macroscopically and histologically.

Small intestinal manifestations

Jejunal and ileal involvement is demonstrated in about 50% of CCS patients.

Large intestinal manifestations

The colon is almost universally affected and the rectum is involved in 67% of cases.[106]

Endoscopic and gross appearance

- Compared to other polyposis syndromes, the macroscopic changes of CCS appear much more diffuse (Fig 6.11).

- The presence of mucosal cystic change produces a characteristic granular appearance to the mucosa of the stomach and the intestines and there may be gelatinous-appearing polypoid masses.

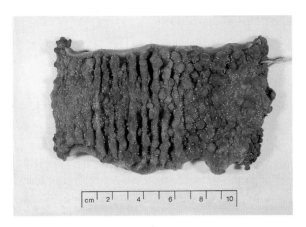

Figure 6.11 – A segment of colon from a patient with Cronkhite–Canada syndrome. Note the low nodular polyps characteristic of the syndrome.

Microscopic features

The morphological features are similar throughout the gut: there is polypoid hyperplasia of the mucosa with cystic dilatation of crypts, flattening of the epithelial surface and oedematous thickening of the lamina propria (Fig 6.12). It has been postulated that this acquired disease is the result of failure of normal epithelial cell proliferative mechanisms throughout ectodermal tissues resulting in hypoplasia of skin and gut epithelium.[107]

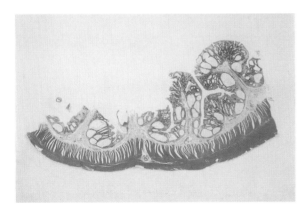

Figure 6.12 – A low power magnification of the colon in a case of Cronkhite–Canada syndrome. There is diffuse cystic dilatation of the mucosa producing polypoid excrescences.

Extra-alimentary manifestations

The cutaneous and other expressions of CCS include alopecia, hyperpigmentation, marked oedema, tetany, glossitis and cataracts.

Malignancy risk

There is now clear evidence of an increased risk of colorectal cancer, at least, in the syndrome: in a recent review, 12% of all the reported cases of the syndrome also suffered from colorectal cancer.[108]

Management

There is no known active treatment for CCS and management of affected patients is merely supportive. The mortality rate is stated to be about 60%.

COWDEN'S SYNDROME

Definition and genetics

Cowden's syndrome is an autosomal dominant familial cancer syndrome in which multiple hamartomas of the skin are associated with polyps of the gastrointestinal tract, central nervous system manifestations and high rates of breast and thyroid malignancy.[109,110]

Synonyms and associations

Multiple hamartoma syndrome, gastrointestinal polyposis with orocutaneous hamartomatosis.

The overlaps, in clinical and molecular terms, with juvenile polyposis have been described previously (see p. 138 above).

Prevalence

Like many polyposis syndromes, Cowden's syndrome is very rare. Curiously, it is named for a family in which the disease occurred.

Molecular pathology

Recent genetic analysis has localised a putative genetic defect for the syndrome to chromosome 10.[110]

Oesophageal manifestations

Papillomatosis of the oropharynx is a characteristic feature.

Gastric, small intestinal and large intestinal manifestations

The polyps are usually dispersed throughout the gastrointestinal tract. They vary greatly in size, number and shape. Some resemble juvenile polyps macroscopically.

Endoscopic and gross appearance

- Because the pathology of the syndrome is not well characterised, no specific endoscopic features have been described (Fig 6.13).

- It should be noted that polyps are only detectable in about 40% of cases.[109]

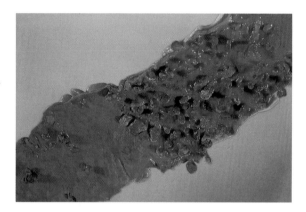

Figure 6.13 – A segment of large intestine in a case of Cowden's syndrome.

Microscopic features

The gastrointestinal polyps are varied histologically and show the features of juvenile polyps, lymphoid polyps, inflammatory polyps, lipomas and ganglioneuromas.

Extra-alimentary manifestations

Patients with Cowden's syndrome show verrucous lesions of the skin, papillomatosis of the lips and oropharynx, *pectus excavatum*, hypoplasia of the jawbones and a high frequency of tumours of the breast and thyroid.

Malignancy risk

High rates of breast and thyroid cancer are notable but no increased risk of gastrointestinal malignancy has been described in the syndrome.[111]

Management

Patients require screening for breast and thyroid disease, as is recommended for Peutz–Jeghers syndrome and FAP, respectively, but management of gastrointestinal involvement is largely supportive only.

CAP (MUCOSAL PROLAPSE) POLYPOSIS

Definition and genetics

The concept of mucosal prolapse being a basic pathological defect causing various heterogeneous presentations is now well accepted.[112] Mucosal prolapse can cause a polypoid mass and, in two situations in the colon, such polyps may be multiple and suggest a polyposis syndrome. Firstly, polypoid mucosal prolapse can be seen as a relatively unusual accompaniment of diverticular disease, on the apices of the crescentic folds.[113] Secondly, cap polyposis is a rare syndrome affecting the sigmoid colon of adults who present with rectal bleeding and mucous diarrhoea.[114,115] Given that cap polyposis is associated with diverticulosis in some cases, it is likely that the two conditions are inter-related.

Synonyms and associations

Mucosal prolapse polyposis.

Some association with diverticular disease of the sigmoid colon.

Prevalence

Exceptionally rare (less than 10 reports in the literature).

Molecular pathology

None described.

Oesophageal and gastric manifestations

None.

Small intestinal manifestations

Granulation tissue polyposis with histological similarities to cap polyposis has been described as a rare complication of carcinoid tumours of the ileum.[116]

Large intestinal manifestations and endoscopic appearance

In cap polyposis, sessile haemorrhagic-appearing polyps are concentrated on the apices of the mucosal folds in the sigmoid colon. There may be associated diverticular disease. This has led to speculation that abnormal sigmoid colonic motility may lead to focal mucosal prolapse at the apices of the crescentic folds and that attendant localised ischaemia produces the characteristic histological appearances.[115] One case has been described after recent pelvic surgery and no motility abnormality was present.[117]

Microscopic features

Cap polyps show the epithelial changes of mucosal prolapse but in addition have a florid granulation tissue component or 'cap' on their surface (Fig 6.14).[114,115]

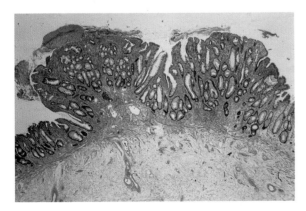

Figure 6.14 – A typical cap polyp. There is a mucosal prolapse polyp with surface ulceration which is 'capped' by exudate.

Extra-alimentary manifestations

None described.

Malignancy risk

None described.

Management

Management is usually supportive, symptoms usually not justifying resection.

BENIGN LYMPHOID POLYPOSIS

Definition and genetics

Benign lymphoid polyposis is a loosely defined condition characterised by multiple lymphoid polyps with benign histological features. It is seen in a variety of situations, most notably in children. It occurs in the terminal ileum of children where it is often a manifestation of immunodeficiency, and in the rectum and less commonly the colon.

In adults other conditions may be characterised by a 'polyposis' due to hyperplastic lymphoid follicles in the intestines. In the duodenum 'lymphoid polyposis' may occur with *Helicobacter*-related pathology. Ulcerative colitis may be accompanied by prominent lymphoid follicular hyperplasia, especially in the rectum. Diversion procto-colitis is characterised by marked nodularity due to hyperplastic lymphoid follicles (see p. 119 in Chapter 5). For the purposes of this discussion, we will confine ourselves to the paediatric diseases of benign lymphoid polyposis of the colorectum and of the ileum.

Synonyms and associations

Terminal ileum – nodular lymphoid hyperplasia.

Prevalence

Not recorded but clinically significant polyposis is exceptionally rare.

Molecular pathology

No known molecular pathology but, in the colon and rectum, the disease represents an exaggerated immune response to viral infection, especially adenovirus and echovirus.[118]

Oesophageal and gastric manifestations

None.

Small and large intestinal manifestations and endoscopic appearance

Innumerable polyps can festoon the intestinal mucosa in these conditions. Apart from being indicators of immuno-deficiency and possible viral infection, the diseases' only significance lies with their mimicry of other polyposis syndromes, most notably FAP.[119] Cases have been recorded in which colectomy has been carried out for this condition in the erroneous belief that multiple polyps equated with FAP.[119] The importance of adequate histological sampling of polyposis syndromes cannot be over-emphasised.

Microscopic features

The polyps show an intact surface mucosa with prominent reactive lymphoid tissue in the underlying submucosa, and often extending into the deep mucosa, as do physiological lymph-glandular complexes.

Extra-alimentary manifestations

None.

Malignancy risk

None for benign lymphoid polyposis of the colorectum. There is a suggestion that some cases of nodular lymphoid hyperplasia of the ileum may precede the development of malignant lymphoma.[120]

Management

In children with rectal or colorectal lymphoid polyposis, response to steroid therapy is often dramatic. Benign lymphoid polyposis of the colon does not appear to have any propensity for malignant change and therefore major surgical resection is not indicated.[121]

MALIGNANT LYMPHOMATOUS POLYPOSIS

Definition and genetics

Malignant lymphomatous polyposis (MLP) is a primary gastrointestinal malignant lymphoma. It is of mantle cell type (Revised European American Lymphoma (REAL) classification), or diffuse centrocytic type (Kiel classification).[122,123]

It is sporadic and no familial tendency has been recorded.

Synonyms and associations

Multiple lymphomatous polyposis. This is the appellation most commonly seen in the medical literature. We believe this term to be tautologous and feel malignant lymphomatous polyposis to be a more apposite title.

Mantle zone lymphoma (REAL classification of malignant lymphoma).

Diffuse centrocytic lymphoma (Kiel classification of malignant lymphoma).

Prevalence

Rare. In one study MLP accounted for 25% of primary large bowel lymphomas.[123] Since these represent only about 4% of all non-Hodgkin lymphomas, MLP certainly accounts for less than 1% of all lymphomas.

Molecular pathology

As with mantle cell lymphomas arising at other sites, notably primary nodal disease, MLP shows *bcl*-1 gene rearrangement and cyclin D1 protein expression, which fully support the theorem that MLP is a gastrointestinal manifestation of mantle cell lymphoma.[124]

Oesophageal manifestations

None.

Gastric manifestations

Gastric involvement certainly does occur but is not as common as intestinal disease.

Small and large intestinal manifestations

In the small intestine, anywhere from the duodenum to the terminal ileum may be involved. A characteristic feature of MLP is massive tumorous involvement of the terminal ileum and caecum. The disease manifests in the small bowel with multiple polyps, which may be especially related to lymphoid aggregates and Peyer's patches. In the colo-rectum, MLP polyps are diffusely distributed but the rectum and ileo-caecal region show the most prominent involvement. In advanced disease, most of the small and large bowel is involved.

Endoscopic and gross appearance

- The polyps of MLP appear to be smooth because of the intact overlying mucosa and usually measure between 0.5 cm and 1 cm.

- The endoscopic appearances are not unlike those of FAP (Fig 6.15).

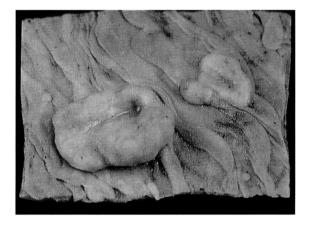

Figure 6.15 – A case of malignant lymphomatous polyposis in the colon in which two polyps are present. The overlying mucosa is intact.

Microscopic features

Although low power histological study shows multinodular lesions, at higher power the characteristic features are a diffuse infiltrate of the lower mucosa and upper submucosa by intermediate-sized lymphoid cells with cleaved nuclei, inconsequential nucleoli and modest amounts of cytoplasm (Fig 6.16). There may be a vague nodularity. The neoplastic mantle cells predominate but there may be an admixture of histiocytes and occasionally granulomas are present in the neoplastic infiltrate. Differentiation from low grade malignant lymphoma of mucosa-associated lymphoid tissue may be difficult, especially on biopsy material. Helpful discriminators between the latter and MLP are the lack of lympho-epithelial lesions and the expression of CD5 and cyclin D1 by the neoplastic mantle cells.[122,123]

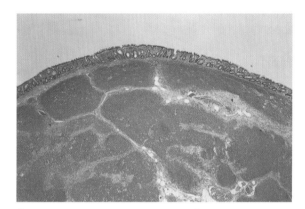

A

B

Figure 6.16 – Although low power histological study (*a*) shows multi-nodular lesions a higher power (*b*) shows that the characteristic features are a diffuse infiltrate of the lower mucosa and upper submucosa by inter-mediate-sized lymphoid cells with cleaved nuclei, inconsequential nucleoli and modest amounts of cytoplasm. There are also bands of hyalinising fibrosis in this example.

Extra-alimentary manifestations

Systemic disease and mantle cell leukaemia are characteristic late features of MLP.[123]

Malignancy risk

MLP is already a malignant condition associated with a considerable adverse prognostic implication.

Management

Because of its multifocal nature, major surgery is usually contraindicated although we have seen a case where the symptoms of colonic involvement (notably excessive mucus loss and electrolyte deficiency) necessitated emergency colectomy. Treatment is primarily by chemotherapy and the prognosis is poor. In one series the majority of patients were dead within 5 years, despite treatment.[123]

INFLAMMATORY FIBROID POLYPOSIS

Definition and genetics

Inflammatory fibroid polyposis (IFP) represents an apparently unique family in which three generations of females have been afflicted by multiple inflammatory fibroid polyps.[125,126] The inheritance, given its specific female occurrence, may yet be autosomal dominant although sex-linked inheritance cannot be ruled out.

Synonyms and associations

The Devon polyposis syndrome.

Prevalence

Excessively rare. Only one Devon UK family, with five cases, all female, in three generations, have been described in the literature.[125,126]

Molecular pathology

Cytogenetic analysis of four affected individuals has been normal.[126] The family has not been agreeable to intensive medical follow-up but identification of the genetic mutation that occasions this syndrome may provide information about the molecular pathogenesis of sporadic IFP.

Oesophageal manifestations

None.

Gastric manifestations

One patient had three polyps in the stomach but otherwise the polyps were confined to the ileum.

Small intestinal manifestations

All five affected cases have had predominant ileal involvement.[126]

Large intestinal manifestations

None.

Endoscopic appearance

- The cases have not been subject to intensive endoscopic investigation largely because of the predominant site of the lesions, the ileum.

Microscopic features

The polyps have all demonstrated the characteristic histological features of inflammatory fibroid polyps (see p. 70 in Chapter 2 and p. 76 in Chapter 4).

Extra-alimentary manifestations

None identified.

Malignancy risk

None identified.

Management

The family has not been amenable to intensive medical follow-up and management of affected cases has been surgical, usually limited right hemicolectomy, when obstructive symptoms have occurred.[126]

REFERENCES

1. Bussey HJR: *Familial Polyposis Coli*. Baltimore, The Johns Hopkins University Press 1975

2. Shepherd NA: Polyps and polyposis syndromes of the intestines. *Curr Diagn Pathol* 1997; **4**: 222–238

3. Gardner EJ: A genetic and clinical study of intestinal polyposis, a predisposing factor for carcinoma of the colon and rectum. *Am J Hum Genet* 1951; **3**: 167–176

4. Turcot J, Despres JP, St Pierre F: Malignant tumors of the central nervous system associated with familial polyposis of the colon: report of two cases. *Dis Colon Rectum* 1959; **2**: 465–468

5. Hamilton SR, Liu B, Parsons RE, *et al*: The molecular basis of Turcot's syndrome. *New Engl J Med* 1995; **332**: 839–847

6. Bulow S: Incidence of associated diseases in familial polyposis coli. *Semin Surg Oncol* 1987; **3**: 84–87

7. Bodmer WF, Bailey CJ, Bodmer J, *et al*: Localization of the gene for familial adenomatous polyposis on chromosome 5. *Nature* 1987; **328**: 614–616

8. Groden J, Thliveris A, Samowitz W, *et al*: Identification and characterization of the familial adenomatous polyposis coli gene. *Cell* 1991; **66**: 589–600

9. Kinzler KW, Nilbert MC, Su L-K, *et al*: Identification of FAP locus genes from chromosome 5q21. *Science* 1991: **253**: 661–664

10. Rubinfeld B, Souza B, Albert I, *et al*: Association of the APC gene product with beta-catenin. *Science* 1993; **262**: 1731–1734

11. Su L-K, Vogelstein B, Kinzler KW: Association of the APC tumor suppressor with catenins. *Science* 1993; **262**: 1734–1737

12. Korinek V, Barker N, Morin PJ, *et al*: Constitutive transcriptional activation by a beta-catenin-Tcf complex in APC-/- colon carcinoma. *Science* 1997; **275**: 1784–1787

13. Morin PJ, Sparks AB, Korinek V, *et al*: Activation of beta-catenin-Tcf signalling in colon cancer by mutations in beta-catenin or APC. *Science* 1997; **275**: 1787–1790

14. Giardiello FM, Brensinger JD, Petersen GM, *et al*: The use and interpretation of commercial APC gene testing for familial adenomatous polyposis. *New Engl J Med* 1997; **336**: 823–827

15. Petersen GM, Brensinger JD: Genetic testing and counseling in familial adenomatous polyposis. *Oncology* 1996; **10**: 89–94

16. van der Luijt RB, Meera Khan P, Vasen HF, *et al*: Germline mutations in the 3′ part of APC exon 15 do not result in truncated proteins and are associated with attenuated adenomatous polyposis coli. *Hum Genet* 1996; **98**: 727–734

17. Giardiello FM, Petersen GM, Piantadosi S, *et al*: APC gene mutations and extraintestinal phenotype of familial adenomatous polyposis. *Gut* 1997; **40**: 521–525

18. Vasen HF, van der Luijt RB, Slors JF, *et al*: Molecular genetic tests as a guide to surgical management of familial adenomatous polyposis. *Lancet* 1996; **348**: 433–435

19. Caspari R, Olschwang S, Friedl W, *et al*: Familial adenomatous polyposis: desmoid tumours and lack of ophthalmic lesions (CHRPE) associated with APC mutations beyond codon 1444. *Hum Mol Genet* 1995; **4**: 337–340

20. Nugent KP, Phillips RK, Hodgson SV, *et al*: Phenotypic expression in familial adenomatous polyposis: partial prediction by mutation analysis. *Gut* 1994; **35**: 1622–1623

21. Watanabe H, Iida M, Iwafuchi M, *et al*: Pathology of gastroenteric lesions in familial adenomatosis coli. In *Hereditary Colorectal Cancer*, Utsunomiya J, Lynch HT (eds). Tokyo, Springer-Verlag 1990: pp. 321–330

22. Park JG, Park KH, Ahn YO, *et al*: Risk of gastric cancer among Korean familial adenomatous polyposis patients: report of three cases. *Dis Colon Rectum* 1992; **35**: 996–998

23. Watanabe H, Enjoji M, Yao T, Ohsato K: Gastric lesions in familial adenomatosis coli. *Hum Pathol* 1978; **9**: 269–283

24. Shepherd NA, Bussey HJR: Polyposis syndromes – an update. In *Gastrointestinal Pathology. Current Topics in Pathology, vol. 81*, Williams GT (ed.). Berlin, Springer-Verlag 1990: pp. 323–351

25. Domizio P, Talbot IC, Spigelman AD, *et al*: Upper gastrointestinal tract pathology in familial adenomatous polyposis. *J Clin Pathol* 1990; **43**: 738–743

26. Spigelman AD, Phillips RKS: The upper gastrointestinal tract. In *Familial Adenomatous Polyposis and Other Polyposis Syndromes*, Phillips RKS, Spigelman AD, Thomson JPS (eds). London, Edward Arnold 1994: pp. 106–127

27. Bulow S, Aim T, Fausa O, *et al*: Duodenal adenomatosis in familial adenomatous polyposis. DAF project. *Int J Colorect Dis* 1995; **10**: 43–46

28. Nugent KP, Spigelman AD, Phillips RK: Life expectancy after colectomy and ileorectal anastomosis for familial adenomatous polyposis. *Dis Colon Rectum* 1993; **36**: 1059–1062

29. Hamilton SR, Bussey HJR, Mendelsohn G, *et al*: Ileal adenomas after colectomy in nine patients with adenomatous polyposis coli/Gardner's syndrome. *Gastroenterology* 1979; **77**: 1252–1257

30. Bertoni G, Sassatelli R, Nigrosoli E, *et al*: First observation of microadenomas in the ileal mucosa of patients with familial adenomatous polyposis and colectomies. *Gastroenterology* 1995; **109**: 374–380

31. Nugent KP, Spigelman AD, Nicholls RJ, *et al*: Pouch adenomas in patients with familial adenomatous polyposis. *Br J Surg* 1993; **80**: 1620.

32. Ziv Y, Fazio VW, Sirimarco MT, *et al*: Incidence, risk factors and treatment of dysplasia in the anal transitional zone after ileal pouch-anal anastomosis. *Dis Colon Rectum* 1994; **37**: 1281–1285

33. Talbot IC: Pathology. In *Familial Adenomatous Polyposis and Other Polyposis Syndromes*, Phillips RKS, Spigelman AD, Thomson JPS (eds). London, Edward Arnold 1994: pp. 15–25

34. Bradburn DM, Gunn A, Hastings AG, *et al*: Histological detection of microadenomas in the diagnosis of familial adenomatous polyposis. *Br J Surg* 1991; **78**: 1394–1395

35. Lynch HT, Smyrk TC, Watson P, *et al*: Hereditary flat adenoma syndrome: a variant of familial adenomatous polyposis? *Dis Colon Rectum* 1992; **35**: 411–421

36. Lipkin M, Blattner WA, Gardner EJ, *et al*: Classification and risk assessment of individuals with familial polyposis, Gardner's syndrome and familial non-polyposis colon cancer from [3H] thymidine labelling patterns in colonic epithelial cells. *Cancer Res* 1984; **44**: 4201–4207

37. Mills SJ, Shepherd NA, Hall PA, *et al*: Proliferative compartment deregulation in the non-neoplastic colonic epithelium of familial adenomatous polyposis. *Gut* 1995; **36**: 391–394

38. Jass JR, Shepherd NA, Maybee JD: Familial adenomatous polyposis. In *An Atlas of Surgical Pathology of the Colon, Rectum and Anus*. Edinburgh, Churchill Livingstone 1989

39. Walsh N, Qizilbash A, Banerjee R, Waugh GA: Biliary neoplasia in Gardner's syndrome. *Arch Pathol Lab Med* 1987; **111**: 76–77

40. Farmer KCR, Hawley PR, Phillips RKS. Desmoid disease. In *Familial Adenomatous Polyposis and Other Polyposis Syndromes*, Phillips RKS, Spigelman AD, Thomson JPS (eds). London, Edward Arnold 1994: pp. 128–142

41. Clark SK, Phillips RK: Desmoids in familial adenomatous polyposis. *Br J Surg* 1996; **83**: 1494–1504

42. Brett MCA, Hershman MJ, Glazer G: Other manifestations of familial adenomatous polyposis. In *Familial Adenomatous Polyposis and Other Polyposis Syndromes*, Phillips RKS, Spigelman AD, Thomson JPS (eds). London, Edward Arnold 1994: pp. 143–160

43. Plain RO, Bussey HJR, Glazer G, Thomson JPS: Adenomatous polyposis: an association with carcinoma of the thyroid. *Br J Surg* 1987; **74**: 377–380

44. Harach HR, Williams GT, Williams ED: Familial adenomatous polyposis associated thyroid carcinoma: a distinct type of follicular cell neoplasm. *Histopathology* 1994; **25**: 549–561

45. Giardiello FM: NSAID-induced polyp regression in familial adenomatous polyposis patients. *Gastroenterol Clin N Am* 1996; **25**: 349–362

46. Piazza GA, Rahm AK, Finn TS, *et al*: Apoptosis primarily accounts for the growth-inhibitory properties of sulindac metabolites and involves a mechanism that is independent of cyclooxygenase inhibition, cell cycle arrest and p53 induction. *Cancer Res* 1997; **57**: 2452–2459

47. McColl I, Bussey HJR, Veale AMC, Morson BC: Juvenile polyposis coli. *Proc R Soc Med* 1964; **57**: 896–897

48. Whitelaw SC, Murday VA, Tomlinson IP, *et al*: Clinical and molecular features of the hereditary mixed polyposis syndrome. *Gastroenterology* 1997; **112**: 327–334

49. Sachatello CR, Griffen WO: Hereditary polypoid diseases of the gastrointestinal tract: a working classification. *Am J Surg* 1975; **129**: 198–203

50. Jass JR: Juvenile polyposis. In *Familial Adenomatous Polyposis and Other Polyposis Syndromes*, Phillips RKS, Spigelman AD, Thomson JPS (eds). London, Edward Arnold 1994: pp. 203–213

51. Sachatello CR, Hahn IS, Carrington CB: Juvenile gastrointestinal polyposis in a female infant. Report of a case and a review of the literature of a recently recognised syndrome. *Surgery* 1974; **75**: 107–113

52. Veale AMO, McColl I, Bussey HJR, Morson BC: Juvenile polyposis coli. *J Med Genet* 1966; **3**: 5–16

53. Burke AP, Sobin LH: The pathology of Cronkhite–Canada polyps. A comparison to juvenile polyposis. *Am J Surg Pathol* 1989; **13**: 940–946

54. Fargnoli MC, Orlow SJ, Semel-Concepcion J, Bolognia JL: Clinicopathologic findings in the Bannayan–Riley–Ruvalcaba syndrome. *Arch Dermatol* 1996; **132**: 1214–1218

55. Leggett BA, Thomas LR, Knight N, *et al*: Exclusion of APC and MCC as the gene defect in one family with familial juvenile polyposis. *Gastroenterology* 1993; **105**: 1313–1316

56. Jacoby RF, Schlack S, Sekhon G, Laxova R: Del (10) (q22.3q24.1) associated with juvenile polyposis. *Am J Med Genet* 1997; **70**: 361–364

57. Jacoby RF, Schlack S, Cole CE, *et al*. A juvenile polyposis tumor suppressor locus at 10q22 is deleted from non-epithelial cells in the lamina propria. *Gastroenterology* 1997; **112**: 1398–1403

58. Subramony C, Scott-Conner CE, Skelton D, Hall TJ: Familial juvenile polyposis. Study of a kindred: evolution of polyps and relationship to gastrointestinal carcinoma. *Am J Clin Pathol* 1994; **102**: 91–97

59. Wu TT, Rezai B, Rashid A, *et al*: Genetic alterations and epithelial dysplasia in juvenile polyposis syndrome and sporadic juvenile polyps. *Am J Pathol* 1997; **150**: 939–947

60. Hizawa K, Iida M, Yao T, *et al*: Juvenile polyposis of the stomach: clinicopathological features and its malignant potential. *J Clin Pathol* 1997; **50**: 771–774

61. Watanabe A, Nagashima H, Motoi M, Ogawa K: Familial juvenile polyposis of the stomach. *Gastroenterology* 1979; **77**: 148–151

62. Jarvinen HJ, Sipponen P: Gastroduodenal polyps in familial adenomatous and juvenile polyposis. *Endoscopy* 1986; **18**: 230–234

63. Stoltenberg RL, Madsen JA, Schlack SC, *et al*: Neoplasia in ileal pouch mucosa after total proctocolectomy for juvenile polyposis: report of a case. *Dis Colon Rectum* 1997; **40**: 726–730

64. Scott-Conner CE, Hausmann M, Hall TJ, *et al*: Familial juvenile polyposis: patterns of recurrence and implications for surgical management. *J Am Coll Surg* 1995; **181**: 407–413

65. Jass JR, Williams CB, Bussey HJR, Morson BC: Juvenile polyposis: a precancerous condition. *Histopathology* 1988; **13**: 619–630

66. Grigioni WF, Alampi G, Martinelli G, Piccaluga A: Atypical juvenile polyposis. *Histopathology* 1981; **5**: 361–376

67. Jarvinen H, Franssila KO: Familial juvenile polyposis coli: increased risk of colorectal cancer. *Gut* 1984; **25**: 792–800

68. Desai DC, Neale KF, Talbot IC, *et al*: Juvenile polyposis. *Br J Surg* 1995; **82**: 14–17

69. Stemper TJ, Kent TH, Summers RW: Juvenile polyposis and gastrointestinal carcinoma. *Ann Int Med* 1975; **83**: 639–646

70. Murday V, Slack J: Inherited disorders associated with colorectal cancer. *Cancer Surv* 1989; **8**: 139–157

71. Giardiello FM, Hamilton SR, Kern SE, *et al*: Colorectal neoplasia in juvenile polyposis or juvenile polyps. *Arch Dis Childhood* 1991; **66**: 971–975

72. Heiss KF, Schaffner D, Ricketts RR, Winn K: Malignant risk in juvenile polyposis coli: increasing documentation in the pediatric age group. *J Pediatr Surg* 1993; **28**: 1188–1193

73. Rodriguez-Bigas MA, Penetrante RB, Herrera L, Petrelli NJ: Intraoperative small bowel enteroscopy in familial adenomatous and familial juvenile polyposis. *Gastrointest Endosc* 1995; **42**: 560–564

74. Peutz JLA. [Very remarkable case of familial polyposis of mucous membrane of intestinal tract and nasopharynx accompanied by peculiar pigmentations of skin and mucous membrane.] *Ned Maandschr Geneesk* 1921; **1**: 134–146

75. Jeghers H, McKusick VA, Katz KH: Generalised intestinal polyposis and melanin spots of the oral mucosa, lips and digits. A syndrome of diagnostic significance. *New Engl J Med* 1949; **241**: 993–1005, 1031–1036

76. Spigelman AD, Phillips RKS: Peutz–Jeghers syndrome. In *Familial Adenomatous Polyposis and Other Polyposis Syndromes*, Phillips RKS, Spigelman AD, Thomson JPS (eds). London, Edward Arnold 1994: pp. 188–202

77. Tomlinson IP, Olschwang S, Abelovitch D, *et al*: Testing candidate loci on chromosomes 1 and 6 for genetic linkage to Peutz–Jeghers' disease. *Ann Hum Genet* 1996; **60**: 377–384

78. Hemminki A, Tomlinson I, Markie D, *et al*: Localization of a susceptibility locus for Peutz–Jeghers syndrome to 19p using comparative genomic hybridization and targeted linkage analysis. *Nat Genet* 1997; **15**: 87–90

79. de Facq L, de Sutter J, de Man M, *et al*: A case of Peutz–Jeghers syndrome with nasal polyposis, extreme iron deficiency anemia, and hamartoma-adenoma transformation: management by combined surgicsal and endoscopic approach. *Am J Gastroenterol* 1995; **90**: 1330–1332

80. Reid JD: Intestinal carcinoma in the Peutz–Jeghers syndrome. *J Am Med Assoc* 1974; **229**: 833–834

81. Defago MR, Higa AL, Campra JL, *et al*. Carcinoma in situ arising in a gastric hamartomatous polyp in a patient with Peutz–Jeghers syndrome. *Endoscopy* 1996; **28**: 267

82. Konishi F, Wyse NE, Muto T, *et al*: Peutz–Jeghers polyposis associated with carcinoma of the digestive organs. Report of three cases and review of the literature. *Dis Colon Rectum* 1987; **30**: 790–799

83. Utsunomiya J, Gocho H, Miyanga T, *et al*: Peutz–Jeghers syndrome: its natural course and management. *Johns Hopkins Med J* 1975; **136**: 71–82

84. Kuwano H, Takano H, Sugimachi K: Solitary Peutz–Jeghers type polyp of the stomach in the absence of familial polyposis coli in a teenage boy. *Endoscopy* 1989; **21**: 188–190

85. Shepherd NA, Bussey HJR, Jass JR: Epithelial misplacement in Peutz–Jeghers polyps: a diagnostic pitfall. *Am J Surg Pathol* 1987; **11**: 743–749

86. Kyriakos M, Condon SC: Enteritis cystica profunda. *Am J Clin Pathol* 1978; **69**: 77–85

87. Perzin KH, Bridge MF: Adenomatous and carcinomatous changes in hamartomatous polyps of the small intestine (Peutz–Jeghers syndrome). A report of a case and a review of the literature. *Cancer* 1982; **49**: 971–983

88. Spigelman AD, Murday V, Phillips RKS: Cancer and the Peutz–Jeghers syndrome. *Gut* 1989; **30**: 1588–1590

89. Linos DA, Dozois RR, Dahlin DC, Bartholomew LG: Does Peutz–Jeghers syndrome predispose to gastrointestinal malignancy? A later look. *Arch Surg* 1981; **116**: 1182–1184

90. Hizawa K, Iida M, Matsumoto T, *et al*: Neoplastic transformation arising in Peutz–Jeghers polyposis. *Dis Colon Rectum* 1993; **36**: 953–957

91. Scully RE: Sex cord tumour with annular tubules. A distinctive ovarian tumour of the Peutz–Jeghers syndrome. *Cancer* 1970; **25**: 1107–1121

92. Young RH, Welch WR, Dickersin GR, Scully RE: Ovarian sex cord tumor with annular tubules. Review of 74 cases including 27 with Peutz–Jeghers syndrome and four with adenoma malignum of the cervix. *Cancer* 1982; **50**: 1384–1402

93. Dozois RR, Judd ES, Dahlin DC, Bartholomew L: The Peutz–Jeghers syndrome. Is there a predisposition to the development of intestinal malignancy? *Arch Surg* 1969; **98**: 509–547

94. Giardiello FM, Welsh SB, Hamilton SR, *et al*: Increased risk of cancer in Peutz–Jeghers syndrome. *New Engl J Med* 1987; **316**: 1511–1514

95. Williams GT, Arthur JF, Bussey HJR, Morson BC: Metaplastic polyps and polyposis of the large intestine. *Histopathology* 1980; **4**: 155–170

96. Spjut HJ, Estrada RG: The significance of epithelial polyps of the large bowel. *Pathol Ann* 1977; **12**: 147–170

97. Bengoechea O, Martinez-Penuela JM, Larrinaga B, *et al*: Hyperplastic polyposis of the colorectum and adenocarcinoma in a 24-year-old man. *Am J Surg Pathol* 1987; **11**: 323–327

98. McGann BG: A case of metaplastic polyposis of the colon associated with focal adenomatous change and metachronous adenocarcinoma. *Histopathology* 1988; **13**: 700–702

99. Joregensen H, Mogensen AM, Svendsen LB: Hyperplastic polyposis of the large bowel. Three cases and a review of the literature. *Scand J Gastroenterol* 1996; **31**: 825–830

100. Jeevaratnam P, Cottier DS, Browett PJ, *et al*: Familial giant hyperplastic polyposis predisposing to colorectal cancer: a new hereditary bowel cancer syndrome. *J Pathol* 1996; **179**: 20–25

101. Sumner HW, Wasserman NF, McClain CJ: Giant hyperplastic polyposis of the colon. *Dig Dis Sci* 1981; **26**: 85–89

102. Shepherd NA: Inverted hyperplastic polyposis of the colon. *J Clin Pathol* 1993; **46**: 56–60

103. Kusunoki M, Fujita S, Sakanoue Y, *et al*: Disappearance of hyperplastic polyposis after resection of rectal cancer. *Dis Colon Rectum* 1991; **34**: 829–831

104. Williams GT: Metaplastic polyposis. In *Familial Adenomatous Polyposis and Other Polyposis Syndromes*, Phillips RKS, Spigelman AD, Thomson JPS (eds). London, Edward Arnold 1994: pp. 174–187

105. Cronkhite LW, Canada WJ: Generalized gastrointestinal polyposis. An unusual syndrome of polyposis, pigmentation, alopecia and onychotrophia. *New Engl J Med* 1955; **252**: 1011

106. Daniel ES, Ludwig SL, Lewin KJ, *et al*: The Cronkhite–Canada syndrome. An analysis of clinical and pathologic features and therapy in 55 patients. *Medicine* 1982; **61**: 293–309

107. Freeman K, Anthony PP, Miller DS, Warin AP: Cronkhite–Canada syndrome: a new hypothesis. *Gut* 1985; **26**: 531–536

108. Nakatsubo N, Wakasa R, Kiyosaki K, *et al*: Cronkhite–Canada syndrome associated with carcinoma of the sigmoid colon: report of a case. *Surg Today* 1997; **27**: 345–348

109. Salem OS, Steck WD: Cowden's disease (multiple hamartoma and neoplasia syndrome). *J Am Acad Dermatol* 1983; **8**: 686–696

110. Nelen MR, Padberg GW, Peeters EA, *et al*: Localization of the gene for Cowden disease to chromosome 10q22-23. *Nat Genet* 1996; **13**: 114–116

111. Haggitt RC, Reid PJ: Hereditary gastrointestinal polyposis syndromes. *Am J Surg Pathol* 1986; **10**: 871–887

112. du Boulay CEH, Fairbrother J, Isaacson PG: Mucosal prolapse syndrome – a unifying concept for solitary ulcer syndrome and allied conditions. *J Clin Pathol* 1983; **36**: 1264–1268

113. Kelly JK: Polypoid prolapsing mucosal folds in diverticular disease. *Am J Surg Pathol* 1991; **15**: 871–878

114. Williams GT, Bussey HJR, Morson BC: Inflammatory 'cap' polyps of the large intestine. *Br J Surg* 1985; **72 supplement**: S133 (Abstract)

115. Campbell AP, Cobb CA, Chapman RW, *et al*: Cap polyposis – an unusual cause of diarrhoea. *Gut* 1993; **34**: 562–564

116. Allibone RO, Hoffman J, Gosney JR, Helliwell TR: Granulation tissue polyposis associated with carcinoid tumours of the small intestine. *Histopathology* 1993; **22**: 475–480

117. Gehenot M, Colombel JF, Wolschies E, *et al*: Cap polyposis occurring in the postoperative course of pelvic surgery. *Gut* 1994; **35**: 1670–1672

118. Atwell JD, Burge D, Wright D: Nodular lymphoid hyperplasia of the intestinal tract in infancy and childhood. *J Pediatr Surg* 1985; **20**: 25–29

119. Berk T, Cohen Z, McLeod RS, Cullen JB: Surgery based on misdiagnosis of adenomatous polyposis. The Canadian Polyposis Registry experience. *Dis Colon Rectum* 1987; **30**: 588–590

120. Matuchansky C, Touchard G, Lemaire M, *et al*: Malignant lymphoma of the small bowel associated with diffuse nodular lymphoid hyperplasia. *New Engl J Med* 1985; **313**: 166–171

121. Benchimol D, Frileux P, Herve de Sigalony JP, Parc R: Benign lymphoid polyposis of the colon. Report of a case in an adult. *Int J Colorectal Dis* 1991; **6**: 165–168

122. Isaacson PG, Maclennan KA, Subbuswamy SG: Multiple lymphomatous polyposis of the gastrointestinal tract. *Histopathology* 1984; **8**: 641–656

123. Shepherd NA, Hall PA, Coates PJ, Levison DA: Primary malignant lymphoma of the colon and rectum: a histopathological and immunohistochemical study of 45 cases with clinicopathological correlations. *Histopathology* 1988; **12**: 235–252

124. Kumar S, Krenacs L, Otsuki T, *et al*: bcl-1 rearrangement and cyclin D1 protein expression in multiple lymphomatous polyposis. *Am J Clin Pathol* 1996; **105**: 737–743

125. Anthony PP, Morris DS, Vowles KDJ: Multiple and recurrent inflammatory fibroid polyps in three generations of a Devon family: a new syndrome. *Gut* 1984; **25**: 854–862

126. Allibone RO, Nanson JK, Anthony PP: Multiple and recurrent inflammatory fibroid polyps in a Devon family ('Devon polyposis syndrome'): an update. *Gut* 1992; **33**: 1004–1005

7

Anal Polyps

I C Talbot and N Y Haboubi

INTRODUCTION

Polyps may arise from outside the anal margin (on the perianal skin) or from within the anal canal, giving a sensation of tenesmus or becoming evident through prolapse onto the perianal surface.

NORMAL STRUCTURE

Normal structure – anatomy

The anal canal extends from the perianal skin to the lower end of the rectum and the upper border of the internal sphincter at the anorectal ring (Fig 7.1). This ring, which lies at the junction of the anal canal and the rectum, contains the upper portion of the internal sphincter, the deep external sphincter and the pubo-rectalis muscles. The dentate (pectinate) line marks the junction between the anal canal and the rectum. A total of 8–16 longitudinal folds, known as the anal columns of Morgagni, cover the underlying blood vessels. They extend from the top end of the anal canal to just below its mid-point. The anal columns connect to one another at the dentate line by the anal valves. These valves form the inner boundaries of small pockets known as the anal crypts of Morgagni. Under the valves, the mucosa joins the hairless skin of the transitional zone in the dentate line. The anal canal mucosa has a glistening wrinkled membranous appearance, which appears discontinuous because of the presence of the anal papillae. These tooth-like raised projections lie on top of the anal columns, extending upwards into the rectum, representing ridges of squamous mucosa contiguous with the rectal mucosa.

The length of the surgical anal canal (which is defined as running from the anorectal ring to the anal verge) is 3–4 cm and is slightly longer in men than in women.

The anal verge marks the junction between the anal canal and the perianal skin.

Normal structure – histology

The anal mucosa contains a mixture of epithelial cell types located in four distinctive zones:[1]

- Colorectal zone. Here the mucosa resembles rectal mucosa, except that the crypts are shorter and more irregular. It is located immediately distal to the rectum and is covered by uninterrupted colorectal mucosa.

- The anal transitional zone. This measures on average 1 cm and macroscopically corresponds to the area of the anal columns. Its distal borders lie at the level of the anal valves and anal sinuses. The epithelial cells form 4–9 layers and contain many cell types. The basal cells appear small and contain nuclei arranged perpendicular to the basement membrane. The surface cells may appear columnar, cuboidal or flattened, often containing a mixture of goblet and non-keratinising squamous cells (Figs 7.2 & 7.3). The cuboidal variant

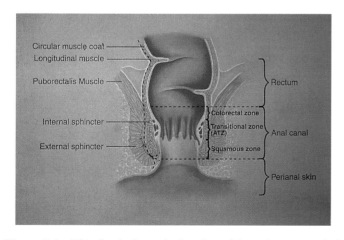

Figure 7.1 – This sketch shows the location of the various anatomical landmarks of the anal canal.

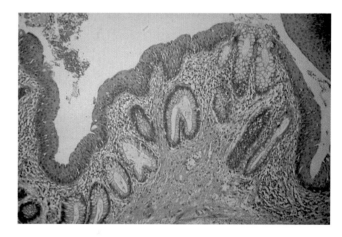

Figure 7.2 – The cloacogenic region of the anal canal. Note the surface epithelium is composed in part of columnar, in part of squamous and in part of transitional epithelium. The surface epithelium overlies rectal type glands.

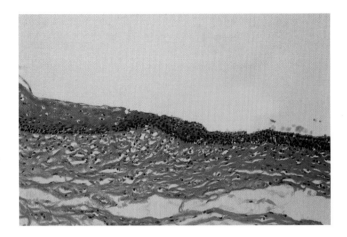

Figure 7.3 – In this field the cloacogenic epithelium is composed of transitional and squamous elements overlying fibrous tissue.

consists of polygonal, flattened cells with horizontally arranged nuclei. The surface cells acquire an umbrella shape with distinct cell borders resembling immature squamous cells, as in squamous metaplasia.

- Squamous zone below the anal columns. This is covered by uninterrupted non-keratinising squamous epithelium devoid of skin appendages and has a dense fibrotic submucosa.

- The distal zone. This is composed of keratinising squamous epithelium merging with the perianal skin.

Anal glands and ducts

The anal glands originate in the transitional zone from the anal crypts, each having a direct opening into the apex of the anal crypts. In adults, 4–8 anal ducts lie in the anal canal. Each has a short tubular submucosal portion branching into a ramifying glandular pattern. They follow a tortuous course through the lamina propria before penetrating the internal sphincter musculature. They extend through the sphincter (and may reach the perianal fat) generally in an outward and downward direction and occasionally upward above the level of the anal valves. The lining of the anal glands (resembling that of the transitional zone) varies; often appearing squamous at the luminal end, transitional in the middle and simple columnar in the deeper parts. Goblet cells are present in large numbers within the anal ducts, particularly in the terminal portion.

Melanocytes are regularly present in the squamous epithelium below the dentate line, and with increased numbers peripherally. The pigment is seen more in dark skin. Endocrine and Paneth cells are present in all types of mucosa apart from squamous epithelium.

OLEOGRANULOMAS

Synonyms

Paraffinomas, inflammatory polyps.

Prevalence

These result from material introduced into the anal canal for the treatment of haemorrhoids. They can develop rapidly or they may appear months or even years later.[2]

Macroscopic appearance

- They can present as a firm yellowish-grey tumourous mass.

- They can be mistaken for a tumour.

- They are usually localised to the anal canal just above the dentate line, but may extend into the rectum.

Microscopic features

The histological features reflect the stage of development. In the early stages, there is an acute mixed inflammatory infiltrate with eosinophils and histiocytes associated with fatty droplets. Later, more fibrosis will be seen together with less inflammation.

BARIUM GRANULOMAS

Prevalence

Barium contrast media may extravasate during barium enema through mucosal defects to produce barium granuloma. These again develop in the anorectal area and may simulate carcinoma or haemorrhoids.

The inflammatory response is due to the direct entrance of barium into the mucosal defect due to inflammation, fistula or diverticula.

Microscopic features

The histological features show a foreign body reaction with histiocytes surrounding the barium material. This appears as a fine grey to light green material within and outside macrophages.

WARTS

Synonyms

Condylomata acuminata.

Prevalence

They can occur in both the anal canal and the perianal skin. They develop frequently if there has been anal intercourse.[3] They have increased in prevalence by 50% over the last 20 years.[4]

They are seen mostly in homosexual men particularly if they are infected with HIV.

They are also seen increasingly in women with cervical, vaginal, vulval and/or perineal warts.

Macroscopic appearance

- There is a wide spectrum of appearances. They can vary from single or multiple growths to lesions that carpet large areas of the anal region.

- They have a characteristic soft, papillary cauliflower-like shape (Fig 7.4) and are of light grey, pink or purple colouration.

Microscopic features

The characteristic histological appearance includes acanthosis resulting in large usually bulbous rete processes, chronic stromal inflammation, hyperkeratosis and variable patchy parakeratosis (Fig 7.5).

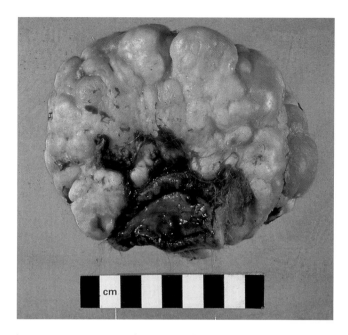

Figure 7.4 – Gross surgical specimen of a perianal condyloma.

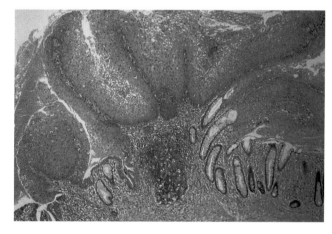

Figure 7.5 – Low magnification histology of a viral-type wart. The lesion is characterised by hyperkeratosis, papillomatosis and acanthosis.

Individual cell keratinisation is often seen and should not be interpreted as a dysplastic feature.

Koilocytotic vacuolation is usual but not invariable and indicates infection with the human papilloma virus (HPV), probably the cause of all of these lesions (Fig 7.6). The nuclei of the affected cells are irregular, hyperchromatic and sometimes multiple. Vacuolation of the epithelial cells alone does not constitute koilocytosis.

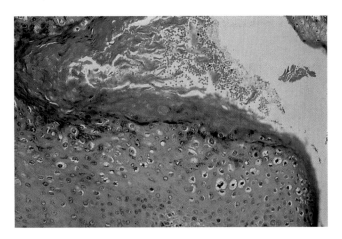

Figure 7.6 – High power view of a viral wart showing koilocytosis, which is typical of viral-type human papilloma virus induced changes.

Biological behaviour and associated conditions

The HPV associated with *condylomata acuminata* is usually Type 6.[5] There is some evidence from studies of proliferating cell nuclear antigen (PCNA) and HPV6 co-expression,[6] that warts are the result of the proliferation of keratinocytes caused by the presence of HPV6.

In individuals with a normal immunological system, keratinocytes that are infected with HPV6 are destroyed by natural killer (NK) cells and by T-lymphocytes activated by intra-epithelial Langerhans cells.[7] This may explain an association between anal warts and smoking.

In contrast to HPV16, 18 and 35, HPV6 seems to have no direct influence in the genesis of neoplasia.[8] This suggests that giant condylomas (Buschke–Lowenstein tumour), which have also been demonstrated to contain HPV6, are closely related, aetiologically, to ordinary condylomas and appear to be condylomas in which excessive growth has, for some reason, occurred.

HPV6 can sometimes be present in squamous cell carcinoma, but this appears to indicate an origin from a pre-existing wart, rather than a malignant influence of HPV6 itself. This view accords with evidence that, despite histological similarities between the two entities, differences in HPV and p53 expression suggest that progression from a giant condyloma to a verrucous carcinoma is not a direct process.[8]

Management

The treatment is often difficult, mostly due to re-infection. Local treatment using a cytotoxic chemical, podophyllin, may be used. Scissor excision may be the preferred treatment because it causes few local symptoms. Other methods of treatment have been used with variable success.[9]

INFLAMMATORY CLOACOGENIC POLYPS

Synonyms

Proctitis cystica profunda. Inflammatory myoglandular polyps. (See also Polypoid mucosal prolapse, in Chapter 5, p. 104).

Prevalence

Usually affects patients between the fifth and seventh decades.

Endoscopic appearance

- This is a rounded polypoid mass measuring up to 4 cm (but usually between 2 and 3 cm), formed by a prolapse of a redundant tag of anal transition zone and rectal mucosa downwards through the anus, sometimes occurring with haemorrhoids.[10,11]

- The lesion is often mistaken, clinically, for a neoplasm, either adenoma or even adenocarcinoma because it has a villiform morphology.

Microscopic features (Fig 7.7)

Such polyps consist of a mass of hyperplastic thickened rectal mucosa, covered partly by anal transitional or squamous epithelium and partly by rectal columnar epithelium, frequently with surface ulceration.

The mucosa of the lesion displays the classical features of mucosal prolapse, with elongation and tortuosity of crypts.

Within the lamina propria, smooth muscle fibres extend vertically between the crypts. There is superficial oedema and vascular ectasia.

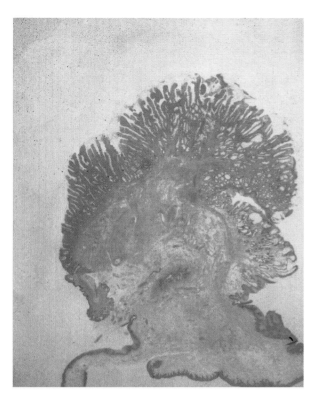

Figure 7.7 – Low power (whole mount) of inflammatory cloacogenic polyp.

The epithelium can appear to be atypical due to hyperplasia.

Sometimes there are displaced glands and cysts in the sub-mucosa; hence the term *proctitis cystica profunda*.[10]

Biological behaviour and associated conditions

These are non-neoplastic, invariably benign, lesions that do not require follow-up.

They may be associated with haemorrhoids and other factors associated with perineal mucosal herniation syndrome and other related conditions.

Management

Simple excision.

PERIANAL SKIN TAGS

Synonyms

Skin tags, sentinel pile.

Prevalence

These are the most frequent anal lesions and are usually clinically trivial or symptomless.

Macroscopic appearance

- They consist of a polypoid mass that ranges in size from under 2 mm to over 1 cm.

Microscopic features

The dermal connective tissue is covered by epidermis-like, mildly keratinising, stratified squamous epithelium. A few skin appendages are usually present. Unless the patient also has Crohn's disease, inflammation is inconspicuous, except at the point of continuity with a neighbouring fissure/ulcer.

Biological behaviour and associated conditions

They are often associated with localised inflammatory diseases (such as fissure or fistula) and are what is left after healing of the damaged skin; from which circumstance they derive their alternative name of 'sentinel pile'.

They can be a source of discomfort especially if they are associated with active inflammation as in Crohn's disease.[12]

Management

Conservative treatment and, if necessary, simple local excision.

FIBROUS POLYPS OF THE ANAL CANAL

Prevalence

These are usually found and removed if the patient is also undergoing treatment of remaining haemorrhoids.

153

Macroscopic appearance

- These are firm, sessile, nodules that form as the end-result of organisation after thrombosis of a haemorrhoid.

- They measure up to 2 cm in diameter.

- They have a firmer core than the surrounding tissue and a denser fibrous stroma than perianal tags.

Microscopic features

They are covered (mainly) by poorly keratinised, stratified, squamous epithelium derived from the transitional zone of the anal canal.

Biological behaviour and associated conditions

They are usually symptomless.

HAEMORRHOIDS

Synonyms

Piles.

Prevalence

This is one of the commonest ailments that affects human beings, but it is very difficult to give an accurate statistical assessment because a significant percentage do not come to hospital for treatment.

There are normally three concentrically arranged groups of anorectal vascular cushions, situated beneath the mucosa of the anal canal. Their normal function is probably to contribute to continence by filling the residual luminal space of the anal canal. During defaecation they empty and collapse. Haemorrhoids are the prolapse of these cushions, usually all three together.

This is a common phenomenon, but what causes it is unknown (apart from the obvious forces of gravity and passage of stool).[13] If the prolapse extends down as far as the verge of perianal skin, a distressing painful incontinent state develops.

Macroscopic appearance

- Surgically excised haemorrhoids are tags of loose connective tissue containing large sinusoidal blood vessels.

Microscopic features

Loose connective tissue containing vascular spaces together with scanty bands of smooth muscle, covered by a mixture of rectal and anal mucosa and perianal skin.

One or more of the vascular spaces may be thrombosed, with varying degrees of organisation and recanalisation.

The surface epithelium is rarely ulcerated and haemorrhoids are rarely inflamed.

Inflammatory cloacogenic polyps frequently accompany haemorrhoids when they extend through the anus, suggesting that the prolapse which produces haemorrhoids may be part of a more general process of anal mucosal prolapse. Indeed the overlying rectal-type mucosa shares some histological features with solitary ulcer syndrome and related conditions,[14] thus supporting the above theory.

SQUAMOUS CELL CARCINOMA OF THE ANAL CANAL

Synonyms

Epidermoid carcinoma, cloacogenic carcinoma, basaloid carcinoma, transitional carcinoma.

Prevalence

This is a tumour that is seen throughout the world but is more commonly seen in areas of low socio-economic class, particularly parts of Brazil and India.[15]

There is a male to female ratio of 5 : 1.[15]

The incidence correlates with carcinoma of the cervix, penis and vulva, suggesting a common aetiological factor.[15]

It occurs more commonly in male homosexuals.[15]

Macroscopic appearance

- This lesion arises at or around the dentate line in the transitional zone (Fig 7.8).

- Approximately 50% arise in the upper canal and appear as submucosal nodular infiltrates.

Microscopic features

Roughly 50% are non-keratinising and 80% are poorly differentiated (Figs 7.8–7.10).

Verrucous carcinoma is an exophytic, very well differentiated, keratinising variant that is sometimes very difficult to differentiate from giant condyloma.

Biological behaviour and associated conditions

The five year survival rate is approximately 50%.

Prognosis depends on:

Tumour size.

Tumour stage.

Grade.

Depth of invasion. Lesions invading the underlying submucosa or muscle have a 5 year survival rate of up to 90%. By contrast, in those invading the soft tissue outside the muscle the 5 year survival rate drops to approximately 50%. This is based on the size of the tumour, which should be demonstrated both clinically and by imaging. The size, however, can not always be measured accurately using these techniques.

Management

Radiotherapy, with or without chemotherapy, is the primary treatment of choice.[9]

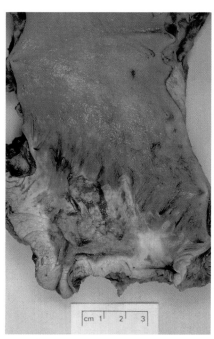

Figure 7.8 – Surgical excision of an anal squamous carcinoma. Note the mixture of papillary and flat configuration.

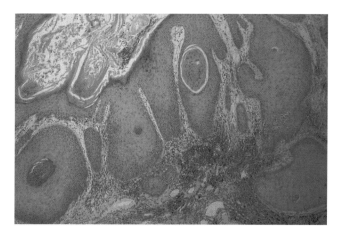

Figure 7.9 – A well differentiated anal squamous cell carcinoma.

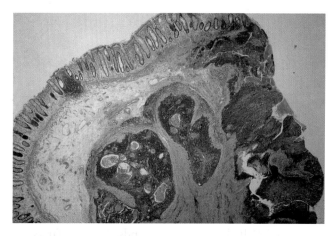

Figure 7.10 – Typical appearance of the so-called basaloid variant of squamous cell carcinoma; here seen infiltrating beneath rectal mucosa. Note the Swiss cheese appearance and the central necrosis of the tumour.

MALIGNANT MELANOMA

Prevalence

Malignant melanoma accounts for 4% of anal canal neo-plasms,[16] 0.048% of all colorectal malignancies and, in Queensland, its incidence relative to cutaneous melanoma is 0.04%.[17]

The mean age of presentation is 66 years and the male:female ratio is 1:1.7.[18] There is evidence from the USA that the incidence has increased and is rising among young men in communities with a high prevalence of HIV infection, such as San Francisco, where there is a bimodal age distribution.[18]

Macroscopic appearance

- These lesions present with bleeding, altered bowel habit or a large polypoid mass prolapsing through the anus, which can be mistaken for haemorrhoids.

- A characteristic feature of these tumours is that they arise in the anal canal but commonly present as anorectal or lower rectal tumours because of anatomical factors. Clinically they often present, therefore, like low rectal adenocarcinomas.

Microscopic features

These are characteristically highly cellular tumours com-posed of solid sheets of cells (Fig 7.11), which have large vesicular nuclei and prominent nucleoli, often with ample eosinophilic cytoplasm but sometimes showing spindle cell forms (mimicking spindle cell squamous carcinoma) or clusters of smaller cells which resemble endocrine tumour (Fig 7.12).

Mitotic figures are numerous. Junctional activity, if present at the lower edge in the anal canal, is diagnostically helpful, but is often obliterated by ulceration.

Melanin pigment is only found in 50% of cases but immunohistochemistry is an important diagnostic aid, since the tumour cells are invariably positive for S100.

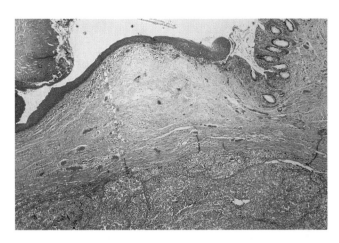

Figure 7.11 – A low power photomicrograph of an anal melanoma occupying the lower part of the field.

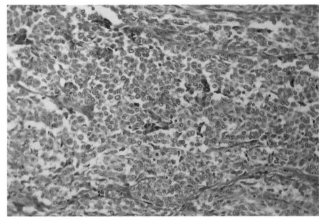

Figure 7.12 – A higher power magnification of the case shown in Fig 7.11. Note the pleomorphic features of the neoplasm.

Biological behaviour and associated conditions

The overall 5 year survival rate in one series was 33%.[16]

Among HIV infected subjects, men have a survival advan-tage, with 1 year survival being 62.8% in men compared with 51.4% in women.

SKIN TUMOURS

The perianal skin can be subject to any of the tumours that arise in the skin at other sites.

Of these, skin appendage tumours, particularly sweat gland tumours, such as nodular hidradenoma, can arise in the anal margin and perianal skin.

Nodular hidradenoma

This typically occurs in middle-aged women and presents as a circumscribed nodule approximately 1 cm in diameter.

Histologically, it shows the highly characteristic appearance of a papillary mass within a cyst-like capsule.

The papillae are lined by a double layer of epithelial cells, the outer layer of which is composed of columnar and cuboidal cells containing PAS-positive mucin.

Anal margin cancer

These are tumours arising below the dentate line but still having a considerable portion of the tumour located in the anal canal. They account for approximately 25% of squamous cell carcinomas. They behave like skin cancer and the prognosis is significantly better than that of anal canal cancer.

OTHER POLYPOIDAL LESIONS

Ectopic tissue

These are types of tissue ectopia that can be seen in the submucosa of the anal canal. Prostatic and salivary gland type tissue have been reported in the rectal mucosa,[19,20] as has gastric heterotopia. They all may present with anal polyps or could even be confused with haemorrhoids.

REFERENCES

1. Normal anatomy of the anus. In *Gastrointestinal Pathology; An Atlas and Text*, 2nd edn, Fenoglio-Preiser CM, Noffsinger A, Stemmermann GN, *et al* (eds). Philadelphia, New York, Lippincott-Raven 1998: pp. 1069–1076

2. Non-neoplastic lesions of the anus. In *Gastrointestinal Pathology; An Atlas and Text*, 2nd edn, Fenoglio-Preiser CM, Noffsinger A, Stemmermann GN, *et al* (eds). Philadelphia, New York, Lippincott-Raven 1998: pp. 1077–1098

3. Peters PK, Mack TM: Patterns of anal carcinoma by gender and marital status in Los Angeles County. *Br J Cancer* 1983; **48:** 624–636

4. Frazer IH, Medley G, Crapper RM, *et al*: Association between anorectal dysplasia, human papilloma virus and human immunodeficiency virus in homosexual men. *Lancet* 1986; **201:** 657–660

5. Rubben A, Spelten B, Albrecht J, Grussendorf-Conen EI: Demonstration of URR-duplication variants of human papilloma virus type 6 in paraffin-embedded tissue sections of one condyloma acuminatum and one Buschke–Lowenstein tumour. *J Pathol* 1994; **174:** 7–12

6. Demeter LM, Stoler MH, Broker TR, Chow LT: Induction of proliferating cell nuclear antigen in differentiated keratinocytes of human papilloma virus-infected lesions. *Hum Pathol* 1994; **25:** 343–348

7. Arany I, Tyring SK: Status of local cellular immunity in interferon-responsive and non-responsive human papilloma virus-associated lesions. *Sexually Trans Dis* 1996; **23:** 475–480

8. Pilotti S, Donghi R, D'Amato L, *et al*: HPV detection and p53 alteration in squamous cell verrucous malignancies of the lower genital tract. *Diagn Mol Pathol* 1993; **2:** 248–256

9. Anal tumours. In *Highlights in Coloproctology*, Schofield PF, Haboubi NY, Martin DF (eds). Springer-Verlag 1993: pp. 148–150

10. Robert PF, Appleman HD: Inflammatory cloacogenic polyp. A unique inflammatory lesion of the anal transitional zone. *Am J Surg Pathol* 1981; **5:** 761–766

11. Chetty R, Bhathal PS, Slavin JL: Prolapse induced inflammatory polyps of the colorectum and anal transitional zone. *Histopathology* 1993; **23:** 63–67

12. Crohn's disease. In *Surgery of the Anus, Rectum and Colon*, 5th edn, Goligher J. (ed.). London, Baillière Tindall 1984: pp. 971–1017

13. Loder PB, Kamm MA, Nicholls RJ, Phillips RK: Haemorrhoids: pathology, pathophysiology and aetiology. *Br J Surg* 1994; **81:** 946–954

14. Kaftan SM, Haboubi NY: Histopathological changes in haemorrhoid associated mucosa and submucosa. *Int J Colorectal Dis* 1995; **10:** 15–18

15. Neoplastic lesions of the anus. In *Gastrointestinal Pathology; An Atlas and Text*, 2nd edn, Fenoglio-Preiser CM, Noffsinger A, Stemmermann GN, *et al* (eds). Philadelphia, New York, Lippincott-Raven 1998: pp. 1099–1128

16. Klas JV, Rothenberger DA, Wong WD, Madoff RD: Malignant tumours of the anal canal: the spectrum of disease, treatment, and outcomes. *Cancer* 1999; **85:** 1686–1693

17. Miller BJ, Rutherford LF, McLeod GR, Cohen JR: Where the sun never shines: anorectal melanoma. *Aust NZ J Surg* 1997; **67:** 846–848

18. Cagir B, Whiteford MH, Topham A, *et al*: Changing epidemiology of anorectal melanoma. *Dis Colon Rectum* 1999; **42:** 1203–1208

19. Morgan MB: Ectopic prostatic tissue of the anal canal. *J Urol* 1992; **147:** 165–166

20. Shindo K, Bacon HE, Holmes EJ: Ectopic gastric mucosa and glandular tissue of salivary type in the anal canal. *Dis Colon Rectum* 1972; **15:** 57–62

8

Preparation and Processing of Polyps

NY Haboubi

INTRODUCTION

Most of the published recommendations for dealing with polyps have been directed toward colonic polyps. We, like others,[1] feel that the preparation and processing of polyps from other sites in the gut would benefit from the application of the same principles.

The appropriate handling of the polyp, which maximises the yield of information that is needed for appropriate management, is the *combined* responsibility of the endoscopist and the pathologist.

The request form should include the following information:

- The endoscopic appearance of the polyp; in particular whether it was sessile or pedunculated.

- The exact site of the polyp

- The size of the polyp; so that the pathologist's report and the endoscopy records can be compared.

- Whether the removal was in one piece *or* in several pieces.

  (a) If the polyp was removed intact and completely, then the diathermy margin should be identified as the resection margin. This margin can be easily recognised as a well defined pale area at one end of the specimen (Figs 8.1 & 8.2). Some workers suggest that this end be identified by the endoscopist with Indian ink or a pin.[2]

  (b) If the polyp was removed in several pieces, it may be impossible to identify the resection margins and consequently the completeness of the excision cannot be commented upon. This information is of paramount importance in the polyp that harbours malignancy. To overcome this problem, it has been suggested that the endoscopist removes and identifies the transected margin separately.[2]

- An indication of whether the removal was complete; with none of the polyp being left behind.

Once the polyp is in the laboratory, proper fixation is mandatory and should not be compromised. Polyps larger than 2 cm may need up to 48 h for formalin to penetrate to the core.[3] Inadequate fixation can lead to: (i) fragmentation of the specimen, which may make meaningful interpretation impossible;[2] (ii) inadequate processing and defects in sections, which may be in areas of highly significant pathology that are no longer present on the slide (Fig 8.3).

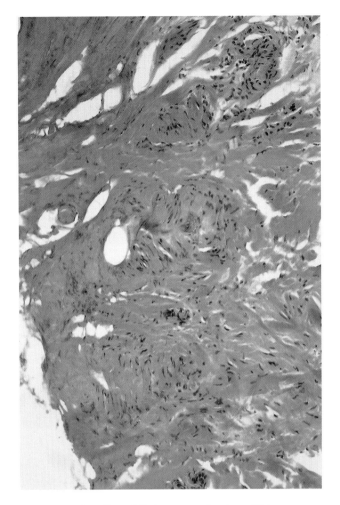

Figure 8.1 – The effect of diathermy on the tissue. This appears as an eosinophilic area of 'mummified' tissue. In this case there is no evidence of tumour in this and other resection margins and the polyp is deemed to have been completely removed.

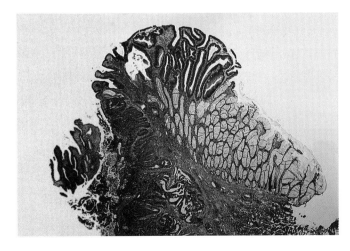

Figure 8.2 – This shows a case of malignant polyp in which the malignant component extends to the (left) resection margin.

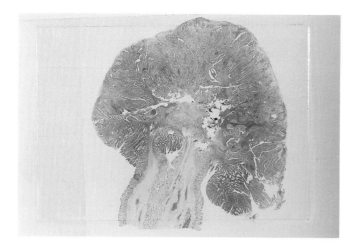

Figure 8.3 – This shows a case of a malignant polyp in which there are tissue defects in the head, neck and the rest of the stalk that were the result of inadequate fixation.

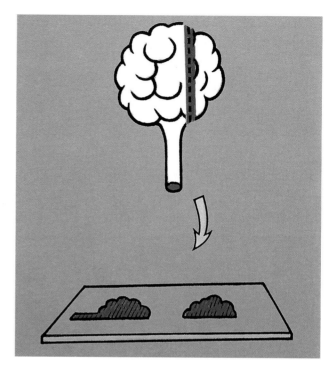

Figure 8.4 – This illustrates one method of trimming stalked polyps.

When the pathologist receives the polyp, the *correct* method of embedding a polyp is very much his/her preference. In the literature there are two main schools of thought concerning polyp processing:

One approach, described by Morson *et al*,[3] is designed to 'produce histological sections in which the normal microanatomical relationship is preserved'. These authors suggest that, if at all possible, the polyp should be embedded whole and on its side and trimming should only be used if necessary. This trimming should be minimal so that the lesion can rest on either side with the intact stalk projecting from one end (Fig 8.4)[1]. These authors further advocate that the polyps should never be cut across if possible. Often various parts of a pedunculated polyp and the muscularis mucosae cannot be clearly identified in the first few levels. Therefore multiple levels and, occasionally, step sectioning are required. It is essential for the surgical pathologist to remember that in order to obtain the correct plane for sectioning it is first necessary to identify the stalk of the polyp.

If the polyp is larger than the standard tissue cassette, then either large cassettes or brass plates should be used and the polyp processed manually if required. After embedding, the block is trimmed to a level where sections can be cut through both the head of the polyp and its stalk in continuity. The correct level can be recognised by the paler colour of the stalk connective tissue compared with that of the head of the polyp.

The various regions of the pedunculated colonic polyp have been defined by Haggitt *et al*[4] as follows: *The head*, which is the area above the junction of the adenoma and the stalk; *the neck*, which is the junction between the adenoma and its stalk; and *the rest of the stalk*. This classification is especially important in the malignant colonic polyp (Fig 8.5).

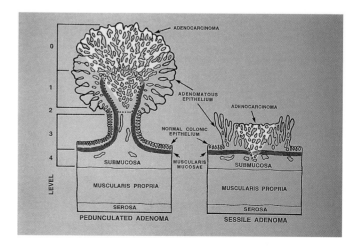

Figure 8.5 – Haggitt's levels of invasion in a malignant polyp.

The second approach advocated by Rosai[5] suggests the following:

(a) For polyps with a short stalk or no stalk, identify the surgical section and cut in half longitudinally.

(b) For polyps with a long stalk (1 cm or more) cut a cross-section of the stalk near the surgical margin and embed separately. Then cut the polyp longitudinally, leaving as long a stalk as will fit in the cassette and embed a representative slice (Fig 8.6).

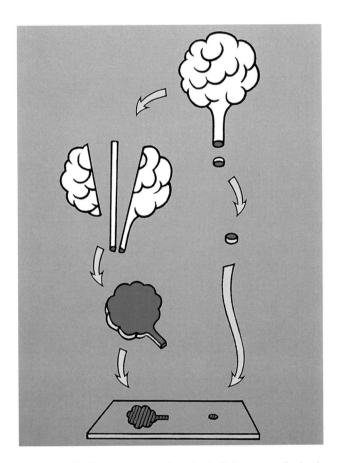

Figure 8.6 – This illustrates a second method of trimming stalked polyps.

(c) If half of the polyp head is over 3 mm, trim to this thickness on the convex side.

The histological report should include the following:

(a) Type of polyp.

(b) Size.

(c) Completeness of excision.

(d) In the case of a malignant colonic polyp the additional information required is:

    (i) The Haggitt level of invasion.
    (ii) Degree of differentiation.
    (iii) Presence of lymphovascular involvement.

These together with the completeness or otherwise of excision will characterise the polyp as a high or low risk malignancy for lymph node involvement and for distant metastasis.

REFERENCES

1. Morson B, Dawson I, Day D, *et al*: Reception and examination of biopsy and surgical specimens. In *Gastrointestinal Pathology*, 3rd edn, Morson B, Dawson I. (eds). Oxford, Blackwell Scientific Publications 1990: pp. 3–7

2. Cooper HS, Deppisch LM, Kahn EI, *et al*: Pathology of the malignant colorectal polyp. *Hum Pathol* 1998; **29:** 15–26

3. Morson BC, Whiteway JE, Jones EA, *et al*: Alimentary tract and pancreas. Histopathology and prognosis of malignant colorectal polyps treated by endoscopic polypectomy. *Gut* 1984; **25:** 437–444

4. Haggitt RC, Glotzbach RE, Soffer EE, Wruble LD: Prognostic factors in colorectal carcinomas arising in adenomas: implications for lesions removed by endoscopic polypectomy. *Gastroenterology* 1985; **89:** 328–336

5. Rosai J: Appendix 4. Guidelines for handling of most common and important surgical specimens. In *Ackerman's Surgical Pathology*, 8th edn, Rosai J (ed.). St Louis, Moseby 1996; pp. 2629–2726

Index